SPRINGER PROTOCOLS HANDBOOKS

T0335416

For further volumes:
http://www.springer.com/series/8623

Animal Coronaviruses

Edited by

Leyi Wang

Animal Disease Diagnostic Laboratory, Ohio Department of Agriculture, Reynoldsburg, OH, USA

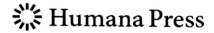 Humana Press

Editor
Leyi Wang
Animal Disease Diagnostic Laboratory
Ohio Department of Agriculture
Reynoldsburg, OH, USA

ISSN 1949-2448   ISSN 1949-2456   (electronic)
Springer Protocols Handbooks
ISBN 978-1-4939-3412-6   ISBN 978-1-4939-3414-0   (eBook)
DOI 10.1007/978-1-4939-3414-0

Library of Congress Control Number: 2016933865

Springer New York Heidelberg Dordrecht London

Printed on acid-free paper

Humana Press is a brand of Springer
Springer Science+Business Media LLC New York is part of Springer Science+Business Media (www.springer.com)

Preface

The first coronavirus, avian infectious bronchitis virus, was isolated from chicken eggs in 1937. Porcine transmissible gastroenteritis virus and mouse hepatitis virus were subsequently identified from pigs and mice, respectively, in the 1940s. In the following decades, while the human coronaviruses were identified in the 1960s, other animal coronaviruses including porcine hemagglutinating encephalomyelitis virus (1962), feline coronavirus (1970), canine coronavirus (1971), bovine coronavirus (1973), turkey coronavirus (1973), porcine epidemic diarrhea virus (1978), and porcine respiratory coronavirus (1984) were also discovered. In order to study coronaviruses, various systems of reverse genetics have been established since 1992 for understanding viral replication, elucidating virus-host interaction and pathogenesis, and developing novel coronavirus vaccines. Because a high-throughput next-generation sequencing technology was unveiled in 2005, its application in virology has advanced a new era of coronavirus discovery. Several emerging animal coronaviruses, such as porcine deltacoronaviruses, therefore, have been identified and characterized. Although there are diverse animal coronavirus species, this handbook is primarily focused on coronaviruses of domestic animals and poultry. This handbook is intended to summarize the currently available technologies that have been developed and utilized to make the progress of coronavirus virology possible. The purpose is to provide the diagnosticians and researchers with practical methodologies and approaches to tackle animal coronaviruses, which cover the conventional immunohistochemistry, virus neutralization, enzyme-linked immunosorbent assays, expression and purification of recombinant viral proteins, and various molecular assays, including conventional and real-time reverse transcription-PCR, reverse genetics methodology, and next-generation sequencing and sequence analyses. Furthermore, it is reasonable to expect that the methodologies and approaches highlighted in this handbook are applicable to other coronavirus species in the *Coronaviridae*.

Reynoldsburg, OH, USA   *Leyi Wang*

Contents

Contributors

MUSTAFA ABABNEH • *Department of Comparative Pathobiology and Animal Disease Diagnostic Laboratory, Purdue University, West Lafayette, IN, USA; Department of Basic Veterinary Medical Sciences, Jordan University of Science and Technology, Irbid, Jordan*

MOHAMED ABDELWAHAB • *Department of Comparative Pathobiology and Animal Disease Diagnostic Laboratory, Purdue University, West Lafayette, IN, USA*

AYDEMIR AKIN • *Department of Comparative Pathobiology and Animal Disease Diagnostic Laboratory, Purdue University, West Lafayette, IN, USA*

AMAURI ALCINDO ALFIERI • *Laboratory of Animal Virology, Department of Veterinary Preventive Medicine, Universidade Estadual de Londrina, Londrina, PR, Brazil*

ALICE FERNANDES ALFIERI • *Laboratory of Animal Virology, Department of Veterinary Preventive Medicine, Universidade Estadual de Londrina (UEL), Londrina, PR, Brazil*

AARON BECKER • *University of Minnesota Genomics Center, University of Minnesota, Saint Paul, MN, USA*

ERICA BICKERTON • *The Pirbright Institute, Compton, Newbury, Berkshire, UK*

ANN BOHAC • *University of Minnesota Genomics Center, University of Minnesota, Saint Paul, MN, USA*

PAUL BRITTON • *The Pirbright Institute, Compton, Newbury, Berkshire, UK*

PATRICK CAMP • *National Veterinary Services Laboratories, Animal and Plant Health Inspection Service, United States Department of Agriculture, Ames, IA, USA*

JIANZHONG CAO • *Department of Comparative Pathobiology and Animal Disease Diagnostic Laboratory, Purdue University, West Lafayette, IN, USA*

WAN-JUNG CHEN • *Department of Comparative Pathobiology and Animal Disease Diagnostic Laboratory, Purdue University, West Lafayette, IN, USA*

YI-NING CHEN • *Department of Comparative Pathobiology and Animal Disease Diagnostic Laboratory, Purdue University, West Lafayette, IN, USA; Department of Bioscience Technology, Chung Yuan Christian University, Chung Li, Taiwan, ROC*

RITA DE CÁSSIA NASSER CUBEL GARCIA • *Departamento de Microbiologia e Parasitologia, Instituto Biomédico, Universidade Federal Fluminense, Niterói, RJ, Brazil*

MING-KUN HSIEH • *Department of Comparative Pathobiology and Animal Disease Diagnostic Laboratory, Purdue University, West Lafayette, IN, USA; Graduate Institute of Microbiology and Public Health, National Chung Hsing University, Taichung, Taiwan, ROC*

KWONIL JUNG • *Food Animal Health Research Program, Ohio Agricultural Research and Development Center, Department of Veterinary Preventive Medicine, The Ohio State University, Wooster, OH, USA*

SARAH M. KEEP • *The Pirbright Institute, Compton, Newbury, Berkshire, UK*

NATHALIE KIN • *Normandie University, Caen, France; EA4655, U2RM, UNICAEN, Caen, France; Department of Virology, University Hospital, Caen, France; Laboratoire de Virologie, Centre Hospitalier Universitaire de Caen, Caen Cedex, France*

MATTI KIUPEL • *Diagnostic Center for Population and Animal Health, College of Veterinary Medicine, Michigan State University, East Lansing, MI, USA; Department of Pathobiology and Diagnostic Investigation, College of Veterinary Medicine, Michigan State University, East Lansing, MI, USA*

TSANG LONG LIN • *Department of Comparative Pathobiology and Animal Disease Diagnostic Laboratory, Purdue University, West Lafayette, IN, USA*

SHENGWANG LIU • *Division of Avian Infectious Diseases, State Key Laboratory of Veterinary Biotechnology, Harbin Veterinary Research Institute, The Chinese Academy of Agricultural Sciences, Harbin, The People's Republic of China*

CHIEN CHANG LOA • *Department of Comparative Pathobiology and Animal Disease Diagnostic Laboratory, Purdue University, West Lafayette, IN, USA; Mylan Pharmaceuticals, Inc., Morgantown, WV, USA*

ROGER K. MAES • *Diagnostic Center for Population and Animal Health, College of Veterinary Medicine, Michigan State University, East Lansing, MI, USA; Department of Pathobiology and Diagnostic Investigation, College of Veterinary Medicine, Michigan State University, East Lansing, MI, USA*

DOUGLAS MARTHALER • *Department of Veterinary Population Medicine, University of Minnesota, Saint Paul, MN, USA*

FABIEN MISZCZAK • *Normandie University, Caen, France; EA4655, U2RM, UNICAEN, Caen, France; Department of Virology, University Hospital, Caen, France; Laboratoire de Virologie, Centre Hospitalier Universitaire de Caen, Caen Cedex, France*

NICHOLE PETERSON • *University of Minnesota Genomics Center, University of Minnesota, Saint Paul, MN, USA*

SUELEE ROBBE-AUSTERMAN • *National Veterinary Services Laboratories, Animal and Plant Health Inspection Service, United States Department of Agriculture, Ames, IA, USA*

TAKEHISA SOMA • *Veterinary Diagnostic Laboratory, Marupi Lifetech Co., Ltd., Ikeda, Osaka, Japan; Department of Veterinary Internal Medicine, School of Veterinary Science, Osaka Prefecture University, Izumisano, Osaka, Japan*

TOD STUBER • *National Veterinary Services Laboratories, Animal and Plant Health Inspection Service, United States Department of Agriculture, Ames, IA, USA*

JUNFENG SUN • *Division of Avian Infectious Diseases, State Key Laboratory of Veterinary Biotechnology, Harbin Veterinary Research Institute, The Chinese Academy of Agricultural Sciences, Harbin, The People's Republic of China*

ELISABETE TAKIUCHI • *Department of Veterinary Sciences, Universidade Federal do Paraná, (UFPR) - Setor Palotina, Palotina, PR, Brazil*

GERGELY TEKES • *Institute of Virology, Faculty of Veterinary Medicine, Justus-Liebig-University Giessen, Giessen, Germany*

VINCENT TESSON • *Normandie University, Caen, France; EA4655, U2RM, UNICAEN, Caen, France; Department of Virology, University Hospital, Caen, France; Laboratoire de Virologie, Centre Hospitalier Universitaire de Caen, Caen Cedex, France*

ASTRID VABRET • *Normandie University, Caen, France; EA4655, U2RM, UNICAEN, Caen, France; Department of Virology, University Hospital, Caen, France; Laboratoire de Virologie, Centre Hospitalier Universitaire de Caen, Caen Cedex, France*

RAMESH VEMULAPALLI • *Department of Comparative Pathobiology, College of Veterinary Medicine, Purdue University, West Lafayette, IN, USA*

LEYI WANG • *Animal Disease Diagnostic Laboratory, Ohio Department of Agriculture, Reynoldsburg, OH, USA*

ANNABEL G. WISE • *Diagnostic Center for Population and Animal Health, College of Veterinary Medicine, Michigan State University, East Lansing, MI, USA*

CHING CHING WU • *Department of Comparative Pathobiology and Animal Disease Diagnostic Laboratory, Purdue University, West Lafayette, IN, USA; School of Veterinary Medicine, National Taiwan University, Taipei, Taiwan, ROC*

YAN ZHANG • *Animal Disease Diagnostic Laboratory, Ohio Department of Agriculture,*

Part I

Introduction

Chapter 1

Animal Coronaviruses: A Brief Introduction

Leyi Wang and Yan Zhang

Abstract

Coronaviruses (CoVs) are single-stranded positive-sense enveloped RNA viruses. Among RNA viruses, CoVs have the largest genome. CoVs infect diverse animal species including domestic and wild animals. In this chapter, we provide a brief review on animal CoVs by discussing their receptor, host specificity, reverse genetics, and emerging and re-emerging porcine CoVs.

Key words Animal coronavirus, Receptor, Reverse genetics, Porcine coronavirus

1 Classification

Coronaviruses (CoVs) belong to *Nidovirales* order, *Coronaviridae* family, *Coronavirinae* subfamily. CoVs contain the largest RNA genome, ranging from 25 to 33 kilobases in length [1]. Based on the phylogenetic analysis, CoVs are classified into four genera, alpha, beta, gamma, and delta CoVs. CoVs of each genus are found in diverse animal species including horses, cows, pigs, dogs, cats, birds, and ferrets (Fig. 1) and cause respiratory, enteric, hepatitic, renal, neurological, and other diseases. It still remains unclear how CoVs of each species evolve and correlate but different evolution models have been proposed. In 2007, the first evolution model on CoV was proposed that bat CoVs serve as gene sources of all CoVs [2]. However, evidence accumulated during the following 2 years seems not to support this hypothesis [1]. Another evolution model was then proposed that bat CoV serves gene sources of alpha and beta CoV while bird CoV serves gene sources of gamma and delta CoV [3].

2 Receptor and Host

Upon receptor binding and membrane fusion, CoVs enter cells and replicate in the cytoplasm. CoVs in each genus utilize different receptors for attachment. For *Alphacoronavirus* genus, porcine,

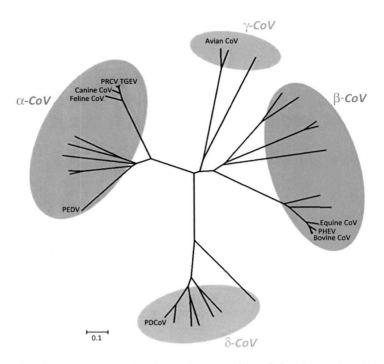

Fig. 1 Phylogenetic tree constructed on the basis of the whole-genome sequences by using the neighbor-joining method in the MEGA software package, version 6.05 (www.megasoftware.net) shows major animal coronaviruses in each genus. *CoV* coronavirus, *TGEV* transmissible gastroenteritis virus, *PRCV* porcine respiratory coronavirus, *PEDV* porcine epidemic diarrhea virus, *PHEV* porcine hemagglutinating encephalomyelitis virus, *PDCoV* porcine deltacoronavirus

feline, and canine CoVs utilize amino peptidase (APN) as receptors (Table 1). N-terminal domain of S1 of transmissible gastroenteritis virus (TGEV) also binds to sialic acids, responsible for TGEV enteric tropism which porcine respiratory coronavirus (PRCV) lacks due to deletion of N-terminal domain [4]. In addition to porcine APN, porcine epidemic diarrhea virus (PEDV) recognizes sugar coreceptor *N*-acetylneuraminic acid [5]. For *Betacoronavirus genus*, both porcine hemagglutinating encephalomyelitis coronavirus (PHEV) and bovine CoV utilize 5-*N*-acetyl-9-*O*-acetylneuraminic acid (Neu5,9Ac2) as entry receptors [6–8] (Table 1). Unlike other porcine CoVs, PHEV is a highly neurotropic virus causing porcine encephalomyelitis. The neural cell adhesion molecule (NCAM) has been identified as a receptor for PHEV [9]. A further study reported that a small fragment (258-amino acid) of 5′ spike protein of PHEV is responsible for interaction with NCAM [10]. For *Gammacoronavirus genus*, infectious bronchitis virus (IBV) recognizes sialic acid as attachment receptor while turkey CoV uses non-sialylated type 2 poly-LacNAc [11, 12] (Table 1). Porcine deltacoronavirus (PDCoV) is a newly identified CoV causing diarrhea in pigs and its receptors remain unknown [13].

Table 1
Animal coronaviruses, tropism, and receptors

Genus	Virus species	Tropism	Receptor	Note
Alpha	TGEV	Respiratory, enteric infection	Aminopeptidase N	Sialic acid
	PRCV	Respiratory infection	Aminopeptidase N	
	PEDV	Enteric infection	Aminopeptidase N	*N*-acetylneuraminic acid
	FIPV	Respiratory, enteric, hepatitis, neurological infection	Aminopeptidase N	
	FECV	Enteric infection	Aminopeptidase N	
	CCoV	Enteric infection	Aminopeptidase N	
Beta	PHEV	Respiratory, enteric, neurological infection	Neu5,9Ac2 NCAM	
	Bovine CoV	Respiratory, enteric infection	Neu5,9Ac2	
	Equine CoV	Enteric infection	ND	
Gamma	IBV	Respiratory, hepatitis, renal infection	Sialic acid	
	TCoV	Enteric infection	Poly-LacNAc	
Delta	PDCoV	Enteric infection	ND	

CoV coronavirus, *TGEV* transmissible gastroenteritis virus, *PRCV* porcine respiratory coronavirus, *PEDV* porcine epidemic diarrhea virus, *FIPV* feline infectious peritonitis virus, *FECV* feline enteric coronavirus, *CCoV* canine coronavirus, *PHEV* porcine hemagglutinating encephalomyelitis virus, *IBV* infectious bronchitis virus, *TCoV* turkey coronavirus, *PDCoV* porcine deltacoronavirus, *Neu5,9Ac2* 5-N-acetyl-9-O-acetylneuraminic acid, *NCAM* neural cell adhesion molecule, *ND* not determined

3 Reverse Genetics

Reverse genetics is a useful approach to study viral pathogenicity and transmission. Two different technologies, targeted recombination and full-length cDNA, are used to develop reverse genetics of CoVs. Due to the largest RNA genome of CoVs, initially there were challenges to develop full-length cDNA clones. Therefore, the first reverse genetics system for CoV was developed by using the targeted recombination in 1990s [14]. Targeted recombination-based reverse genetics system has been developed for TGEV and FIPV [15, 16]. However, some disadvantages including inability to modify replicase region of viral genome prevent its wide applications. Subsequently, full-length cDNA-based reverse genetics system was developed. Three methods including in vitro ligation, bacterial artificial chromosome (BAC) vector, and vaccinia virus have been used to rescue CoVs from full-length cDNA. The full-length cDNA-based reverse genetics system was developed for TGEV by rescuing infectious clones using either in vitro ligation or BAC vector approach [17, 18]. In the case of IBV, the reverse genetics system was established using in vitro ligation or vaccinia virus [19, 20]. Full-length cDNA-based reverse genetics system of BAC vector or vaccinia viral vector was also developed for FIPV

[21, 22]. Recently, targeted recombination and BAC vector-based full-length cDNA methods have been applied to PEDV [23, 24]. The availability of different reverse genetics systems will promote research on the molecular biology and pathogenicity of CoVs. The reverse genetics also holds a promising approach to develop vaccine candidates against PEDV and other porcine coronaviruses.

4   Emerging and Re-emerging Porcine CoVs

There are five porcine CoVs, TGEV, PRCV, PEDV, PHEV, and PDCoV. Porcine CoVs cause respiratory (PRCV), enteric (TGEV, PEDV, and PDCoV), and neurological diseases (PHEV) in pigs and threaten swine industries worldwide. Since 2013, porcine CoVs are emerging and re-merging in different countries, raising concerns on how to control and eradicate them from pigs.

4.1   PEDV

PEDV was first identified in Belgium in 1970s [25]. Following that, PEDV has spread throughout many countries of Europe in 1980s and 1990s. Since 2000, it has only been sporadically detected in Europe, but frequently reported in Asian countries including China, South Korea, and Thailand [26]. Since 2010, a highly pathogenic PEDV emerged in China and caused significant economic problems [27, 28]. In May 2013, this PEDV was detected in the USA and Canada soon after and caused severe economic loss to the swine industry [29]. More recently, it has re-emerged in several European countries including Germany, France, and Belgium [30–33]. These data indicate a pandemic outbreak of this PEDV.

Currently, there are at least two different strains, classical and variant, circulating in the USA. The variant strain (OH851) was first identified in January of 2014 in Ohio [34]. In comparison with the initial classical strain, the variant strain contains three deletions, one insertion, and lots of point mutations in the first 1170 nt of 5′ S1 region with only 89 % nucleotide similarity; by contrast, there is 99 % nucleotide similarity in the remaining genome [34]. Phylogenetic analysis of the full-length genome showed both classical and variant strains cluster together belonging to genogroup 2; however, the phylogenetic analysis of the spike gene indicates that the variant strain is more closely related to genogroup 1 but distantly related with the US classical strain [34]. The variant strain is relatively underestimated in the USA due to that the real-time RT-PCR assay commonly used in the diagnostic laboratories could not distinguish between them. By utilizing primers targeting on the conserved regions of S1 but probes targeting on the variable regions of S1, a differential real-time RT-PCR assay has been developed to detect and differentiate variant from classical PEDV [35]. Currently, the variant strain was also reported in Germany, Belgium, France, Portugal, Japan, and Taiwan [30–33, 36]. It remains unclear about the origin of the variant strain, but the field evidence suggests that the variant strain could evolve from the classical strain through mutations or recombination.

4.2 PDCoV

PDCoV was first identified in a surveillance study in Hong Kong in 2012, in which 17 out of 169 fecal swab samples were positive for PDCoV; however, its role as a pathogen was not reported [3]. In February 2014, PDCoV was identified in the pigs with clinical diarrheal symptoms in the US Ohio state. The complete genome analysis of two Hong Kong strains (HKU15-155, -44) and one Ohio strain (OH1987) reveals that there is a high nucleotide similarity among them [13]. Further analysis of strains of nine US states and Hong Kong indicates that there is a single genotype circulating in the field [37, 38]. Subsequently, PDCoV was also detected in Canada, South Korea, and Mainland China [39]. Genomic analysis showed that PDCoV from South Korea closely correlated with US strains and HKU15-44 without any nucleotide deletion in the genome whereas three strains from Mainland China have a three-nucleotide deletion in either S gene or 3' untranslated region (UTR) and are different from HKU15-155 which has both deletions in S and 3' UTR. It still remains unknown about how the different PDCoV strains evolve in pigs and is critical to monitor the virus using the whole-genome sequencing. Recently, the PDCoV has been successfully cultured and isolated in ST or LLC-PK cell lines [40].

For the newly identified pathogens, the important question to answer is to fulfill the Koch's postulate. Animal challenge experiments recently conducted on different ages of either gnotobiotic or conventional pigs showed that PDCoV isolated from clinical samples reproduced the diarrheal diseases. Jung et al. demonstrated that 11- to 14-day-old gnotobiotic pigs inoculated with two strains of PDCoV (OH-FD22 and OH-FD100) showed severe diarrhea and vomiting symptoms and shed the highest amount of viruses at 24 or 48 h post-inoculation, consistent with the onset of clinical signs [41]. Histopathologic observation indicates that the jejunum and ileum are the major sites of PDCoV infection [41]. Similarly, Ma et al. showed that a plaque-purified PDCoV strain (Michigan/8977/2014) reproduced the diarrheal disease in 10-day-old gnotobiotic pigs and cause severe villous atrophy of small intestines; however, the amount of viral shedding in the conventional 10-day-old pigs challenged with the same strain does not correlate with the severity of diarrhea [42]. On the contrary, Chen et al. reported that severity of diarrhea in the 5-day-old conventional piglets inoculated with another plaque-purified PDCoV (USA/IL/2014) correlated with the viral shedding [43]. These differences may result from the different ages of piglets or different PDCoV strains used in the experiments. We also observed that piglets naturally infected with PDCoV developed similar macroscopic and microscopic lesions in small intestines to those in experimental piglets, but less severe than those caused by PEDV (unpublished data).

4.3 PRCV

PRCV, the TGEV deletion variant, was first identified in Belgium in 1980s [44] and then has been detected in other parts of Europe, Asia, and North America [45–48]. Unlike that TGEV replicates in both intestinal and respiratory tracts, PRCV almost exclusively replicates in the respiratory tract due to a 621–681 nt deletion in the S gene. PRCV infection causes mild or subclinical respiratory diseases or contributes to the porcine respiratory disease complex. Recently, we have identified a new PRCV variant strain (OH7269) from the clinical samples. OH7269 has 648 nt deletion in the 5′ S1 region and 3 nt deletion at position 2866–2868 nt of S gene. In addition, two new deletions were observed in the intergenic region of S and ORF3a, and ORF3a [49]. Genomic similarity between TGEV and PRCV has greatly complicated the differential diagnosis. The real-time RT-PCR assay with primers and probes targeting on the conserved region of N and other genes could not distinguish between TGEV and PRCV [50]. Accordingly, a nested RT-PCR assay targeting on the spike (S) 1 region of both viruses was developed [51]. In addition to the S gene, ORF3a and 3b are mostly studied and different insertion and deletion patterns were reported [52]. By amplifying and sequencing the complete genome of ORF3a and ORF3b for 20 PRCV strains, we were able to identify several new PRCV variants with new insertions/deletions in intergenic region of S and ORF3a, ORF3a, and ORF3b (unpublished data). These variants cause mild respiratory diseases either alone or together with swine influenza virus or porcine reproductive and respiratory syndrome virus, indicating that PRCV continuously evolves in the pigs.

5 Conclusion

Since severe acute respiratory syndrome (SARS) outbreak in 2003, there has been a significant increase on coronavirus research. Several human and animal coronaviruses including Middle East respiratory syndrome (MERS) CoV and PDCoV have been identified [53]. It is highly likely that more emerging and re-emerging CoVs are to be identified in the future owing to the availability of new technologies including next-generation sequencing. Future research efforts should focus on studying how CoVs adapt to new hosts, identifying intermediate hosts, and monitoring evolution of CoVs.

References

1. Woo PC, Lau SK, Huang Y, Yuen KY (2009) Coronavirus diversity, phylogeny and interspecies jumping. Exp Biol Med 234:1117–1127

2. Vijaykrishna D, Smith GJ, Zhang JX, Peiris JS, Chen H, Guan Y (2007) Evolutionary insights into the ecology of coronaviruses. J Virol 81:4012–4020

3. Woo PC, Lau SK, Lam CS, Lau CC, Tsang AK, Lau JH, Bai R, Teng JL, Tsang CC, Wang M, Zheng BJ, Chan KH, Yuen KY (2012) Discovery of seven novel Mammalian and

avian coronaviruses in the genus deltacoronavirus supports bat coronaviruses as the gene source of alphacoronavirus and betacoronavirus and avian coronaviruses as the gene source of gammacoronavirus and deltacoronavirus. J Virol 86:3995–4008

4. Schultze B, Krempl C, Ballesteros ML, Shaw L, Schauer R, Enjuanes L, Herrler G (1996) Transmissible gastroenteritis coronavirus, but not the related porcine respiratory coronavirus, has a sialic acid (N-glycolylneuraminic acid) binding activity. J Virol 70:5634–5637

5. Liu C, Tang J, Ma Y, Liang X, Yang Y, Peng G, Qi Q, Jiang S, Li J, Du L, Li F (2015) Receptor usage and cell entry of porcine epidemic diarrhea coronavirus. J Virol 89:6121–6125

6. Krempl C, Schultze B, Herrler G (1995) Analysis of cellular receptors for human coronavirus OC43. Adv Exp Med Biol 380:371–374

7. Schultze B, Gross HJ, Brossmer R, Klenk HD, Herrler G (1990) Hemagglutinating encephalomyelitis virus attaches to N-acetyl-9-O-acetylneuraminic acid-containing receptors on erythrocytes: comparison with bovine coronavirus and influenza C virus. Virus Res 16:185–194

8. Schultze B, Gross HJ, Brossmer R, Herrler G (1991) The S protein of bovine coronavirus is a hemagglutinin recognizing 9-O-acetylated sialic acid as a receptor determinant. J Virol 65:6232–6237

9. Gao W, He W, Zhao K, Lu H, Ren W, Du C, Chen K, Lan Y, Song D, Gao F (2010) Identification of NCAM that interacts with the PHE-CoV spike protein. Virol J 7:254

10. Dong B, Gao W, Lu H, Zhao K, Ding N, Liu W, Zhao J, Lan Y, Tang B, Jin Z, He W, Gao F (2015) A small region of porcine hemagglutinating encephalomyelitis virus spike protein interacts with the neural cell adhesion molecule. Intervirology 58:130–137

11. Wickramasinghe IN, de Vries RP, Weerts EA, van Beurden SJ, Peng W, McBride R, Ducatez M, Guy J, Brown P, Eterradossi N, Grone A, Paulson JC, Verheije MH (2015) Novel receptor specificity of avian gammacoronaviruses causing enteritis. J Virol 89:8783–8792

12. Winter C, Schwegmann-Wessels C, Cavanagh D, Neumann U, Herrler G (2006) Sialic acid is a receptor determinant for infection of cells by avian Infectious bronchitis virus. J Gen Virol 87:1209–1216

13. Wang L, Byrum B, Zhang Y (2014) Detection and genetic characterization of deltacoronavirus in pigs, Ohio, USA, 2014. Emerg Infect Dis 20:1227–1230

14. Koetzner CA, Parker MM, Ricard CS, Sturman LS, Masters PS (1992) Repair and mutagenesis of the genome of a deletion mutant of the coronavirus mouse hepatitis virus by targeted RNA recombination. J Virol 66:1841–1848

15. Haijema BJ, Volders H, Rottier PJ (2003) Switching species tropism: an effective way to manipulate the feline coronavirus genome. J Virol 77:4528–4538

16. Sanchez CM, Izeta A, Sanchez-Morgado JM, Alonso S, Sola I, Balasch M, Plana-Duran J, Enjuanes L (1999) Targeted recombination demonstrates that the spike gene of transmissible gastroenteritis coronavirus is a determinant of its enteric tropism and virulence. J Virol 73:7607–7618

17. Almazan F, Gonzalez JM, Penzes Z, Izeta A, Calvo E, Plana-Duran J, Enjuanes L (2000) Engineering the largest RNA virus genome as an infectious bacterial artificial chromosome. Proc Natl Acad Sci U S A 97:5516–5521

18. Yount B, Curtis KM, Baric RS (2000) Strategy for systematic assembly of large RNA and DNA genomes: transmissible gastroenteritis virus model. J Virol 74:10600–10611

19. Casais R, Thiel V, Siddell SG, Cavanagh D, Britton P (2001) Reverse genetics system for the avian coronavirus infectious bronchitis virus. J Virol 75:12359–12369

20. Youn S, Leibowitz JL, Collisson EW (2005) In vitro assembled, recombinant infectious bronchitis viruses demonstrate that the 5a open reading frame is not essential for replication. Virology 332:206–215

21. Balint A, Farsang A, Zadori Z, Hornyak A, Dencso L, Almazan F, Enjuanes L, Belak S (2012) Molecular characterization of feline infectious peritonitis virus strain DF-2 and studies of the role of ORF3abc in viral cell tropism. J Virol 86:6258–6267

22. Tekes G, Hofmann-Lehmann R, Stallkamp I, Thiel V, Thiel HJ (2008) Genome organization and reverse genetic analysis of a type I feline coronavirus. J Virol 82:1851–1859

23. Jengarn J, Wongthida P, Wanasen N, Frantz PN, Wanitchang A, Jongkaewwattana A (2015) Genetic manipulation of porcine epidemic diarrhea virus (PEDV) recovered from a full-length infectious cDNA clone. J Gen Virol 96:2206–2218

24. Li C, Li Z, Zou Y, Wicht O, van Kuppeveld FJ, Rottier PJ, Bosch BJ (2013) Manipulation of the porcine epidemic diarrhea virus genome using targeted RNA recombination. PLoS One 8:e69997

25. Pensaert MB, de Bouck P (1978) A new coronavirus-like particle associated with diarrhea in swine. Arch Virol 58:243–247

26. Song D, Park B (2012) Porcine epidemic diarrhoea virus: a comprehensive review of molecular epidemiology, diagnosis, and vaccines. Virus Genes 44:167–175

27. Bi J, Zeng S, Xiao S, Chen H, Fang L (2012) Complete genome sequence of porcine epidemic diarrhea virus strain AJ1102 isolated from a suckling piglet with acute diarrhea in China. J Virol 86:10910–10911

28. Li W, Li H, Liu Y, Pan Y, Deng F, Song Y, Tang X, He Q (2012) New variants of porcine epidemic diarrhea virus, China, 2011. Emerg Infect Dis 18:1350–1353

29. Stevenson GW, Hoang H, Schwartz KJ, Burrough ER, Sun D, Madson D, Cooper VL, Pillatzki A, Gauger P, Schmitt BJ, Koster LG, Killian ML, Yoon KJ (2013) Emergence of Porcine epidemic diarrhea virus in the United States: clinical signs, lesions, and viral genomic sequences. J Vet Diagn Invest 25:649–654

30. Grasland B, Bigault L, Bernard C, Quenault H, Toulouse O, Fablet C, Rose N, Touzain F, Blanchard Y (2015) Complete genome sequence of a porcine epidemic diarrhea s gene indel strain isolated in France in December 2014. Genome Announc 3:pii: e00535-15

31. Hanke D, Jenckel M, Petrov A, Ritzmann M, Stadler J, Akimkin V, Blome S, Pohlmann A, Schirrmeier H, Beer M, Hoper D (2015) Comparison of porcine epidemic diarrhea viruses from Germany and the United States, 2014. Emerg Infect Dis 21:493–496

32. Stadler J, Zoels S, Fux R, Hanke D, Pohlmann A, Blome S, Weissenbock H, Weissenbacher-Lang C, Ritzmann M, Ladinig A (2015) Emergence of porcine epidemic diarrhea virus in southern Germany. BMC Vet Res 11:142

33. Theuns S, Conceicao-Neto N, Christiaens I, Zeller M, Desmarets LM, Roukaerts ID, Acar DD, Heylen E, Matthijnssens J, Nauwynck HJ (2015) Complete genome sequence of a porcine epidemic diarrhea virus from a novel outbreak in Belgium, January 2015. Genome Announc 3:pii: e00506-15

34. Wang L, Byrum B, Zhang Y (2014) New variant of porcine epidemic diarrhea virus, United States, 2014. Emerg Infect Dis 20:917–919

35. Wang L, Zhang Y, Byrum B (2014) Development and evaluation of a duplex real-time RT-PCR for detection and differentiation of virulent and variant strains of porcine epidemic diarrhea viruses from the United States. J Virol Methods 207:154–157

36. Chiou HY, Huang YL, Deng MC, Chang CY, Jeng CR, Tsai PS, Yang C, Pang VF, Chang HW (2015) Phylogenetic analysis of the spike (S) gene of the new variants of porcine epidemic diarrhoea virus in Taiwan. Transbound Emerg Dis. doi:10.1111/tbed.12357

37. Wang L, Byrum B, Zhang Y (2014) Porcine coronavirus HKU15 detected in 9 US states, 2014. Emerg Infect Dis 20:1594–1595

38. Wang L, Zhang Y, Byrum B (2014) Complete genome sequence of porcine coronavirus HKU15 strain IN2847 from the United States. Genome Announc 2:pii:e00291–14

39. Lee S, Lee C (2014) Complete genome characterization of Korean Porcine deltacoronavirus strain KOR/KNU14-04/2014. Genome Announc 2:pii:e01191–14

40. Hu H, Jung K, Vlasova AN, Chepngeno J, Lu Z, Wang Q, Saif LJ (2015) Isolation and characterization of porcine deltacoronavirus from pigs with diarrhea in the United States. J Clin Microbiol 53:1537–1548

41. Jung K, Hu H, Eyerly B, Lu Z, Chepngeno J, Saif LJ (2015) Pathogenicity of 2 porcine deltacoronavirus strains in gnotobiotic pigs. Emerg Infect Dis 21:650–654

42. Ma Y, Zhang Y, Liang X, Lou F, Oglesbee M, Krakowka S, Li J (2015) Origin, evolution, and virulence of porcine deltacoronaviruses in the United States. mBio 6:e00064

43. Chen Q, Gauger P, Stafne M, Thomas J, Arruda P, Burrough E, Madson D, Brodie J, Magstadt D, Derscheid R, Welch M, Zhang J (2015) Pathogenicity and pathogenesis of a United States porcine deltacoronavirus cell culture isolate in 5-day-old neonatal piglets. Virology 482:51–59

44. Pensaert M, Callebaut P, Vergote J (1986) Isolation of a porcine respiratory, non-enteric coronavirus related to transmissible gastroenteritis. Vet Q 8:257–261

45. Chae C, Kim O, Min K, Choi C, Kim J, Cho W (2000) Seroprevalence of porcine respiratory coronavirus in selected Korean pigs. Prev Vet Med 46:293–296

46. Elazhary Y, Jabrane A, Talbot BG (1992) Porcine respiratory coronavirus isolated from young piglets in Quebec. Vet Rec 130:500

47. Have P (1990) Infection with a new porcine respiratory coronavirus in Denmark: serologic differentiation from transmissible gastroenteritis virus using monoclonal antibodies. Adv Exp Med Biol 276:435–439

48. Wesley RD, Woods RD, Hill HT, Biwer JD (1990) Evidence for a porcine respiratory coronavirus, antigenically similar to transmissible gastroenteritis virus, in the United States. J Vet Diagn Invest 2:312–317

49. Wang L, Zhang Y (2015) Genomic characterization of a new PRCV variant, United States, 2014. Transbound Emerg Dis. doi:10.1111/tbed.12400

50. Kim SH, Kim IJ, Pyo HM, Tark DS, Song JY, Hyun BH (2007) Multiplex real-time RT-PCR for the simultaneous detection and quantification of transmissible gastroenteritis virus and

porcine epidemic diarrhea virus. J Virol Methods 146:172–177

51. Kim L, Chang KO, Sestak K, Parwani A, Saif LJ (2000) Development of a reverse transcription-nested polymerase chain reaction assay for differential diagnosis of transmissible gastroenteritis virus and porcine respiratory coronavirus from feces and nasal swabs of infected pigs. J Vet Diagn Invest 12:385–388

52. Kim L, Hayes J, Lewis P, Parwani AV, Chang KO, Saif LJ (2000) Molecular characterization and pathogenesis of transmissible gastroenteri-

tis coronavirus (TGEV) and porcine respiratory coronavirus (PRCV) field isolates co-circulating in a swine herd. Arch Virol 145:1133–1147

53. de Groot RJ, Baker SC, Baric RS, Brown CS, Drosten C, Enjuanes L, Fouchier RA, Galiano M, Gorbalenya AE, Memish ZA, Perlman S, Poon LL, Snijder EJ, Stephens GM, Woo PC, Zaki AM, Zambon M, Ziebuhr J (2013) Middle East respiratory syndrome coronavirus (MERS-CoV): announcement of the Coronavirus Study Group. J Virol 87:7790–7792

Part II

Conventional Technologies

Chapter 2

Immunohistochemical Staining for Detection of Porcine Epidemic Diarrhea Virus in Tissues

Kwonil Jung

Abstract

Porcine epidemic diarrhea virus (PEDV), a member of the genus *Alphacoronavirus*, has resulted in significant economic losses in the European, Asian, and North American swine industries in previous years. PEDV infection causes acute diarrhea/vomiting, dehydration, and high morbidity and mortality in seronegative neonatal piglets. In this chapter, materials and methods for performing immunohistochemistry (IHC) for the detection of PEDV antigens in frozen or formalin-fixed, paraffin-embedded (FFPE) tissues are provided. In IHC of frozen tissues where viral antigens are well preserved, the use of specific antibodies labeled with fluorescence dyes provides excellent advantages and convenience, resulting in high sensitivity and specificity of IHC and reduction of operation time. In IHC of FFPE tissues where tissue or cell morphology is well preserved, the use of specific antibodies labeled with enzymes, such as alkaline phosphatase, also gives rise to significant advantages in defining the correlation of viral antigens with histopathologic lesions. PEDV antigens in frozen tissues are visualized as green staining in the cytoplasm of infected cells by fluorescent dyes conjugated with antibodies when activated by exciting light of a specific wavelength under a fluorescence microscope. In FFPE tissues, PEDV antigens are visualized as red staining in the cytoplasm of infected cells by the deposition of the substrate chromogen, Fast Red.

Key words Porcine epidemic diarrhea virus, PEDV, Immunohistochemistry, Diagnosis, Detection, Pig, Virus

1 Introduction

The family *Coronaviridae* can be divided into four genera: *Alphacoronavirus*, *Betacoronavirus*, *Gammacoronavirus*, and *Deltacoronavirus*. Porcine epidemic diarrhea virus (PEDV), a member of the genus *Alphacoronavirus*, causes acute diarrhea, vomiting, dehydration, and high mortality in neonatal piglets, resulting in significant economic losses, initially only seen in the European and Asian swine industries over the last three decades. Recently, however, PEDV was first reported in the USA in May 2013 in Iowa [1]. Since then, the virus has rapidly spread nationwide [2] and to other countries in North America, including Canada and Mexico. The PED epidemic in the USA, from April

Leyi Wang (ed.), *Animal Coronaviruses*, Springer Protocols Handbooks,
DOI 10.1007/978-1-4939-3414-0_2, © Springer Science+Business Media New York 2016

2013 to present, has led to a substantial loss of piglets (more than 10 % of US swine population). Because of similar clinical and pathogenic features between PEDV and another *Alphacoronavirus*, transmissible gastroenteritis virus (TGEV), or a *Deltacoronavirus*, porcine deltacoronavirus (PDCoV), differential laboratory tests are required for their diagnosis [3–5]. Reverse transcription-polymerase chain reaction (RT-PCR) or quantitative RT-PCR (qRT-PCR) is useful for the rapid differential diagnosis; however, detection of viral antigens in tissues is essential for confirming each viral infection.

Viral antigens in frozen, fixed cells, or tissues can be detected by immunohistochemistry (IHC) (or immunohistochemical staining) using specific antibodies labeled with fluorescent dyes, such as Alexa Fluor®488 and fluorescein isothiocyanate (FITC), or enzymes, such as alkaline phosphatase (AP) and peroxidase. Immunofluorescence (IF) staining is the first immunohistochemical staining method but is still widely used in veterinary and medical diagnosis. With fundamentality of antigen-antibody and antibody-antibody binding reactions, antigens are visualized by fluorescent dyes conjugated with antibodies when activated by an exciting light of a specific wavelength (499–519 nm for Alexa Fluor®488 and 494–521 nm for FITC), under a fluorescence microscope. Due to the high sensitivity, specificity, and convenience in using Alexa Fluor®488 in frozen tissues, this chapter details an IF staining method for the rapid and precise detection of PEDV antigens in PEDV-infected, frozen tissues, contributing to verification of the tissue sites of PEDV replication in infected pigs. A combination of PEDV-specific anti-sera as antigen detection antibody and secondary antibody conjugated with Alexa Fluor®488 is applied in the IF staining method. However, because of suboptimal conditions of tissue or cell morphology in frozen tissues, this staining method limits investigation of the correlation of PEDV antigens with histopathologic lesions.

To compensate for the limitation of IF staining in frozen tissues, additional IHC staining method using enzyme-labeled antibodies, i.e., immunoenzymological staining, in formalin-fixed, paraffin-embedded (FFPE) tissues is also provided in this chapter. After adding a substrate of enzyme, such as Fast Red, it generates insoluble particles that can be localized in cells or tissues under light microscope. Compared to the IF staining in frozen tissues, the IHC in FFPE tissues has more accurate localization of antigens with a better contrast ratio, contributing to defining the correlation of PEDV antigen-positive cells with severity of histopathologic lesions caused by PEDV, such as intestinal villous atrophy.

Only one serotype of PEDV has been reported from different countries [4]. There has been no evidence of cross-reactivity of PEDV with TGEV [6, 7]. The use of hyperimmune anti-sera or polyclonal antibodies against PEDV in IHC staining is likely able to detect geographically different strains of PEDV and differentiate them from TGEV in tissues [8, 9], but with a potential disadvantage of inducing background or false signals. To improve the sensitivity and specificity of IHC for the detection of PEDV antigens in tissues, the use of monoclonal antibodies to structural proteins of PEDV, such as spike (S) or membrane (M) protein, has been preferred [10, 11]. Prior to their application on the tissues, potential cross-reactivity of monoclonal antibodies to TGEV and PDCoV can be tested by more sensitive assays, such as enzyme-linked immunosorbent assay, immunoblotting, and immunoprecipitation, compared to IHC.

Tissue tropism of PEDV is related to the expression of aminopeptidase N (APN), a 150 kDa glycosylated transmembrane protein identified as the cellular receptor, on porcine small intestinal villous enterocytes [12]. PEDV-infected enterocytes rapidly undergo acute necrosis, leading to marked villous atrophy in the small but not large intestine [10]. In PEDV-infected nursing pigs, major histologic lesions include acute diffuse, severe atrophic enteritis, and mild vacuolation of superficial epithelial cells and subepithelial edema in cecum and colon [8–10, 13]. PEDV antigens are observed mainly in villous enterocytes of the small (duodenum to ileum) and large intestines (except rectum) [1, 8, 10]. Occasionally, a few PEDV-positive cells were detected in the intestinal crypt cells or the Peyer's patches [1, 8–10]. No lesions were seen in the spleen, liver, lung, kidney, and mesenteric lymph node of orally and/or intranasally infected piglets [8]. Lung tissue of oronasally infected pigs was negative for PEDV antigen [1, 8–10]. PEDV antigens were not detected in other major organs, such as the pylorus, tonsils, liver, and kidneys. However, a recent study reported the replication of PEDV in swine pulmonary macrophages in vitro and in vivo [14].

Epidemic PEDV strains are highly enteropathogenic and acutely infect villous epithelial cells of the entire small and large intestines, but the jejunum and ileum are the primary sites of infection. To detect PEDV antigen in tissues and evaluate the pathogenicity of PEDV strains in pigs, the jejunum and ileum are the most critical tissue samples for performing IHC.

2   Materials

2.1   Solutions and Reagents (See Note 1)

1. Primary antibody: Monoclonal antibody 6C8-1 against the spike protein of PEDV strain DR13 kindly provided by Dr. Daesub Song, Korea Research Institute of Bioscience and Biotechnology, Daejeon, Korea.

2. Secondary antibody: Goat anti-mouse IgG antibody conjugated with Alexa Fluor®488 (Invitrogen, Carlsbad, CA, USA) for IF

staining in frozen tissues; goat anti-mouse IgG antibody labeled with alkaline phosphatase (Dako, Glostrup, Denmark) for IHC in FFPE tissues.

IF staining in frozen tissues

1. 10% (w/v) Sucrose solution (pH 7.2).
2. Tissue-Tek® O.C.T™ Compound (Sakura Finetek USA, Inc., Torrance, CA, USA).
3. Liquid nitrogen.
4. 25% (v/v) Acetone in ethanol.
5. Prolong® Gold Antifade Mountant with 4′,6-diamidino-2-phenylindole, dihydrochloride (DAPI) (Invitrogen).
6. 1× Universal Blocking Reagent (Biogenex, Fremont, CA).
7. 1× Phosphate-buffered saline (PBS) (pH 7.4).
8. 1× PBS (pH 7.4) containing Tween 20, 0.1 % (Sigma Aldrich, St. Louis, MO, USA) (PBTS).

IHC in FFPE tissues

1. Xylene (Sigma Aldrich).
2. 100, 95, 70, and 50 % ethanol.
3. 3 % (v/v) glacial acetic acid in deionized water.
4. Proteinase K (Invitrogen, Carlsbad, CA, USA).
5. 1× Universal Blocking Reagent (Biogenex).
6. 1× PBS (pH 7.4).
7. 1× PBS (pH 7.4) containing Tween 20, 0.1 % (Sigma Aldrich, St. Louis, MO, USA) (PBTS).
8. Fast Red (Roche Applied Science, Mannheim, Germany).
9. 0.1 M Tris buffer (pH 8.2).
10. Gill's or Mayer's hematoxylin (Sigma Aldrich).
11. Ultramount Permanent Aqueous Mounting Medium (Dako).

2.2 Equipment/Tools

1. Glass slide-staining dishes or jars.
2. Slide racks and trays.
3. Humidified chamber tray with lid.
4. Adjustable pipettors with tips.
5. Barrier Dako Pen (Dako).
6. 4 °C Refrigerator.
7. 37 °C Incubator.
8. Microscope slides: Superfrost™ Plus Gold Slides (Fisher Scientific, PA, USA).
9. Glass cover slip (Fisher Scientific).

10. Rocker platform shaker.

11. Kimberly-Clark® Kimwipes™ (Kimberly-Clark Corporation, Irving, Texas, USA).

12. Vortex mixer.

IF staining in frozen tissues only

1. –80 °C freezer.

2. Cryostat.

3. Glass dropping pipettes.

4. Fluorescence microscope.

IHC in FFPE tissues only

1. Microtome.

2. 60 °C Oven.

3. 10 ml Syringes.

4. 0.9 µm Syringe filters.

5. Permount permanent mounting media (Fisher Scientific).

6. Light microscope.

3   Methods

3.1   Tissue or Slide Preparation

3.1.1   IF Staining in Frozen Tissues

One to three pieces (2–3 cm per piece) of duodenum, proximal jejunum, mid-jejunum, distal jejunum, ileum, cecum, and colon are collected and perfused with 100–400 ml of 10 % sucrose solution, depending on the size of the immersed tissue. The tissues are trimmed, embedded in OCT compound, and frozen at –80 °C or by liquid nitrogen. Using a cryostat (–20 to –25 °C), tissue sections are cut at 5 to 10 µm thickness and mounted on Superfrost™ Plus Gold Slides. The tissue slides can be stored at –70 to –80 °C for several months. At the beginning of IF staining, the slides are dried for 30 min to 1 h at room temperature (RT). The slides are then fixed and dehydrated with 25 % acetone for 30 min to 1 h at RT.

3.1.2   IHC in FFPE Tissues

FFPE tissue sections are cut at 3 to 4 µm thickness using a microtome and mounted on Superfrost™ Plus Gold Slides in a 55 °C water bath. Tissue slides are dried at 60 °C for 1 h or at 37 °C for 3–4 h or overnight.

3.2   Deparaffinization and Rehydration of Tissue Section Slides (IHC in FFPE Tissues Only)

1. Place slides of FFPE tissues (Sect. 3.1.2) in a slide rack for 15 min at 60 °C.

2. Place the slides in the rack into xylene for 20 min at RT to remove the paraffin.

3. Place the slides in 100 % ethanol for 5 min to rehydrate tissues through a graded ethanol series (100–50 %; the following steps

3–6). Repeat through two changes of fresh 100 % ethanol, 5 min for each.

4. Place the slides in 95 % ethanol for 10 min.

5. Place the slides in 70 % ethanol for 7 min.

6. Place the slides in 50 % ethanol for 7 min.

7. Move the slides into deionized water and wash at RT for 1 min.

8. Move the slides into PBS and immerse at RT for 7 min (*see* **Note 2**).

3.3 Antigen Retrieval (IHC in FFPE Tissues Only)

1. Lay the deparaffinized, rehydrated tissue slides (Sect. 3.2) across a horizontal slide tray or humidified chamber tray.

2. Gently and carefully blot the slides with Kimwipes around the tissue, as well as the non-charged slide surface.

3. Surround the tissue with a hydrophobic barrier using the Dako Pen.

4. Apply 300–500 µl of 3 % glacial acetic acid to quench endogenous alkaline phosphatase and incubate at RT for 20 min.

5. Apply 300–500 µl of proteinase K (100 µg/ml) to the tissue sections with the hydrophobic barrier and incubate at 37 °C for 30 min.

6. Rinse the slides in PBS for 5 min on a rocker platform shaker. Repeat through three changes of fresh PBS, 5 min for each.

3.4 Immunohisto-chemical Staining Protocol

3.4.1 IF Staining in Frozen Tissues

1. Place the fixed, dehydrated tissues (Sect. 3.1.1) in PBS at RT for 5 min to rehydrate (*see* **Note 2**).

2. Lay the tissue slides across a horizontal slide tray or humidified chamber tray.

3. Gently and carefully blot the slides with Kimwipes around the tissue, as well as the non-charged slide surface.

4. Surround the tissue with a hydrophobic barrier using the Dako Pen.

5. Apply 300–500 µl of 1× Universal Blocking Reagent to the tissue within the hydrophobic barrier and incubate at 37 °C for 30 min.

6. Drain the slides and place them on a horizontal surface.

7. Apply the primary antibody (diluted 1:200 in PBTS) enough to cover the tissue section (200–300 µl) and incubate in a humidified chamber at 4 °C overnight (*see* **Note 3**).

8. Rinse the slides gently with PBS on a rocker platform shaker at RT for 5 min. Repeat through three changes of fresh PBS, 5 min for each.

9. Apply the Alexa Fluor®488-labeled secondary antibody (diluted 1:200 in PBTS) enough to cover the tissue section

(200–300 µl) and incubate in a humidified chamber at 37 °C for 1 h (*see* **Note 3**).

10. Rinse the slides gently with PBS on a rocker platform shaker at RT for 5 min. Repeat through three changes of fresh PBS, 5 min for each.

11. Gently blot the slides with Kimwipes around the tissue and place horizontally.

12. Apply 3–5 drops of Prolong® Gold Antifade Mountant (with DAPI) to the tissue section using a glass dropping pipette and immediately put a cover slip on (*see* **Note 4**).

13. The slides are ready to be evaluated under fluorescence microscope. They need to be stored in a dark area until evaluation. PEDV antigens will appear to be green or as fluorescent staining in the cytoplasm of infected cells (Fig. 1). Cell nuclei are stained blue with DAPI.

3.4.2 IHC in FFPE Tissues

1. When antigen retrieval procedure is completed (Sect. 3.3), drop 300–500 µl of 1× Universal Blocking Reagent on the tissue within the hydrophobic barrier and incubate at 37 °C for 30 min.

2. Drain the slides and place them on a horizontal surface.

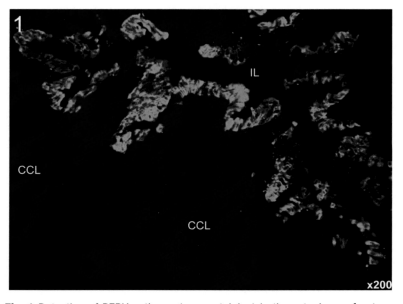

Fig. 1 Detection of PEDV antigens (*green* staining) in the cytoplasm of enterocytes lining atrophied villi by immunofluorescence staining in frozen jejunal tissues using a monoclonal antibody specific for the spike protein of PEDV and secondary antibody conjugated with Alexa Fluor®488. Original magnification ×200. *IL* intestinal lumen, *CCL* crypt cell layer. Nuclei were stained with *blue*-fluorescent 4′,6-diamidino-2-phenylindole, dihydrochloride

3. Apply the primary antibody (diluted 1:200 in PBTS) enough to cover the tissue section (200–300 μl) and incubate in a humidified chamber at 4 °C overnight (*see* **Note 3**).

4. Rinse the slides gently with PBS on a rocker platform shaker at RT for 5 min. Repeat through three changes of fresh PBS, 5 min for each.

5. Apply the AP-labeled secondary antibody (diluted 1:200 in PBTS) enough to cover the tissue section (200–300 μl) and incubate in a humidified chamber at 37 °C for 1 h (*see* **Note 3**).

6. Rinse the slides gently with PBS on a rocker platform shaker at RT for 5 min. Repeat through three changes of fresh PBS, 5 min for each.

7. For step 6, add 1 tablet of Fast Red in 2 ml of 0.1 M Tris buffer (pH 8.2), depending on the number of the tissue sections, and dissolve by a vortex mixer (*see* **Note 5**).

8. Drain the slides and place them on a horizontal surface.

9. Apply the Fast Red solution enough to cover the tissue section (300–500 μl) and incubate in a humidified chamber at RT for 30–60 min (*see* **Note 6**).

10. Place the slides in a rack and rinse well in distilled water. Three changes, 2 min each.

11. Tissue sections are counterstained in a glass dish with Gill's hematoxylin at RT for 10 min.

12. Rinse the slides thoroughly in tap water for 5 min, and move into deionized water.

13. Drain the slides and place them on a horizontal surface.

14. Apply 2–4 drops of Permanent Aqueous Mounting Medium to the tissue section (*see* **Note 7**), and immediately put a cover slip on (*see* **Note 8**).

15. The slides are ready to be evaluated under light microscope. PEDV antigens will appear as a red precipitate in the cytoplasm of infected cells (Fig. 2). Cell nuclei are stained blue with hematoxylin.

4 Notes

1. Use of fresh reagents is recommended. A large amount of washing buffer, 1× PBS, is needed, because complete washing is critical to reduce background and increase true signals.

2. Throughout immunostaining procedures, the tissues should stay rehydrated. Adequate antigen-antibody or antibody-antibody binding reaction is not expected in dried tissues, resulting in poor or weak staining results or a high level of background staining.

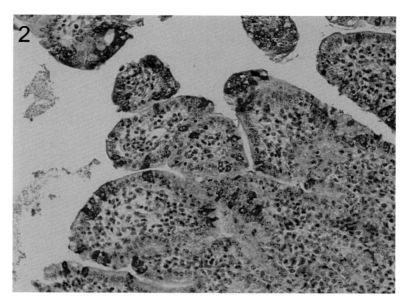

Fig. 2 Detection of PEDV antigens (*red* staining) in the cytoplasm of enterocytes lining atrophied villi by immunohistochemical staining in formalin-fixed, paraffin-embedded jejunal tissues using a monoclonal antibody specific for the spike protein of PEDV and secondary antibody conjugated with alkaline phosphatase. Original magnification ×200. Immunohistochemistry. Fast Red. Gill's hematoxylin counterstaining

It is also critical for a comparative immunostaining study in multiple different tissues.

3. The optimal dilutions of primary and secondary antibodies should be tested and selected in both frozen and FFPE tissue conditions.

4. Instead of plastic pipette tips, the use of glass dropping pipette will reduce the number of bubbles in the mounting medium as applied to the tissue sections.

5. When the Fast Red tablet is completely dissolved, the solution can be filtered via 0.9 μm syringe filter and used to reduce an irregular deposition of Fast Red on the tissues or background.

6. The color development, including intensity of true or false signals, in all tissue slides tested should be frequently monitored under the microscope. Wipe the non-charged slide surface with Kimwipes before putting the tissue slides on the microscope.

7. Gently drop the mounting medium so as not to create bubbles. The mounted slides need to be evaluated as soon as possible, because bubbles can be created spontaneously in the mounted medium.

8. To make the stained slides permanent, a large amount of mounting medium can be applied to the tissues so that the entire section is covered. Place slides horizontally in a 60 °C oven for 30 min to allow the medium to harden. Remove the slides from the oven, and allow them to cool at RT. Dip the slides in xylene and cover slip with permount permanent mounting medium (Fisher Scientific).

Acknowledgements

Salaries and research support were provided by state and federal funds appropriated to the Ohio Agricultural Research and Development Center, The Ohio State University. This work was supported by a grant from the OARDC SEEDS, Grant # OAOH1536.

References

1. Stevenson GW, Hoang H, Schwartz KJ, Burrough EB, Sun D, Madson D, Cooper VL, Pillatzki A, Gauger P, Schmitt BJ, Koster LG, Killian ML, Yoon KJ (2013) Emergence of Porcine epidemic diarrhea virus in the United States: clinical signs, lesions, and viral genomic sequences. J Vet Diagn Invest 25(5):649–654

2. Cima G (2013) Fighting a deadly pig disease. J Am Vet Med A 243(4):467–470

3. Jung K, Saif LJ (2015) Porcine epidemic diarrhea virus infection: Etiology, epidemiology, pathogenesis and immunoprophylaxis. Vet J 204(2):134–143

4. Saif LJ, Pensaert MP, Sestak K, Yeo SG, Jung K (2012) Coronaviruses. In: Zimmerman JJ, Karriker LA, Ramirez A, Schwartz KJ, Stevenson GW (eds) Diseases of swine, 10th edn. Iowa State University, Wiley-Blackwell, pp 501–524

5. Jung K, Hu H, Eyerly B, Lu Z, Chepngeno J, Saif LJ (2015) Pathogenicity of 2 porcine deltacoronavirus strains in gnotobiotic pigs. Emerg Infect Dis 21(4):650–654

6. Hofmann M, Wyler R (1989) Quantitation, biological and physicochemical properties of cell culture-adapted porcine epidemic diarrhea coronavirus (PEDV). Vet Microbiol 20(2):131–142

7. Pensaert MB, Debouck P, Reynolds DJ (1981) An immunoelectron microscopic and immunofluorescent study on the antigenic relationship between the coronavirus-like agent, CV 777, and several coronaviruses. Arch Virol 68(1):45–52

8. Debouck P, Pensaert M, Coussement W (1981) The pathogenesis of an enteric infection in pigs, experimentally induced by the coronavirus-like agent, Cv-777. Vet Microbiol 6(2):157–165

9. Sueyoshi M, Tsuda T, Yamazaki K, Yoshida K, Nakazawa M, Sato K, Minami T, Iwashita K, Watanabe M, Suzuki Y et al (1995) An immunohistochemical investigation of porcine epidemic diarrhoea. J Comp Pathol 113(1):59–67

10. Jung K, Wang Q, Scheuer KA, Lu Z, Zhang Y, Saif LJ (2014) Pathology of US porcine epidemic diarrhea virus strain PC21A in gnotobiotic pigs. Emerg Infect Dis 20(4):662–665

11. Kim O, Chae C, Kweon CH (1999) Monoclonal antibody-based immunohistochemical detection of porcine epidemic diarrhea virus antigen in formalin-fixed, paraffin-embedded intestinal tissues. J Vet Diagn Invest 11(5):458–462

12. Li BX, Ge JW, Li YJ (2007) Porcine aminopeptidase N is a functional receptor for the PEDV coronavirus. Virology 365(1):166–172

13. Coussement W, Ducatelle R, Debouck P, Hoorens J (1982) Pathology of experimental CV777 coronavirus enteritis in piglets. I. Histological and histochemical study. Vet Pathol 19(1):46–56

14. Park JE, Shin HJ (2014) Porcine epidemic diarrhea virus infects and replicates in porcine alveolar macrophages. Virus Res 191:143–152

Chapter 3

Virus Neutralization Assay for Turkey Coronavirus Infection

Yi-Ning Chen, Ching Ching Wu, and Tsang Long Lin

Abstract

Turkey coronavirus (TCoV) infection induces the production of protective antibodies against the sequent exposure of TCoV. Serological tests to determine TCoV-specific antibodies are critical to evaluate previous exposure to TCoV in the turkey flocks and differentiate serotypes from different isolates or strains. A specific virus neutralization assay using embryonated turkey eggs and immunofluorescent antibody assay for determining TCoV-specific neutralizing antibodies is described in this chapter. Virus neutralization titer of turkey serum from turkeys infected with TCoV is the dilution of serum that can inhibit TCoV infection in 50 % of embryonated turkey eggs. Virus neutralization assay for TCoV is useful to monitor the immune status of turkey flocks infected with TCoV for the control of the disease.

Key words Turkey coronavirus, Virus neutralization assay, Turkey embryonated eggs, Immunofluorescence antibody assay

1 Introduction

Turkey coronavirus (TCoV) causes atrophic enteritis in turkeys and belongs to species *Avian coronavirus* of the genus *Gammacoronavirus* in the family *Coronaviridae*. The most closely related coronavirus is infectious bronchitis virus (IBV) causing respiratory disease in chickens. Turkey coronavirus infection induced protective antibody responses because turkeys that survived the infection did not develop clinical signs and TCoV was not detected in their intestines and feces after subsequent exposure to TCoV [1, 2]. Therefore, serological tests can be used to detect previous exposure to TCoV and differentiate the serotypes or strains from different isolates. The TCoV-specific antibodies can be detected by either enzyme-linked immunosorbent assay (ELISA) using TCoV S protein [3, 4], TCoV N protein [5, 6], or IBV virions [7] or immunofluorescent antibody (IFA) assay using intestine sections containing TCoV [8]. Among different serological tests, virus neutralization (VN) assay is the most specific test showing the inhibition of viral infection to target host tissues or cells by protective neutralizing antibodies.

Leyi Wang (ed.), *Animal Coronaviruses*, Springer Protocols Handbooks,
DOI 10.1007/978-1-4939-3414-0_3, © Springer Science+Business Media New York 2016

Without cell culture system available for TCoV, embryonated turkey eggs are used for VN assay of TCoV. Because TCoV infection usually does not cause embryonic death, IFA assay [4, 8] or real-time RT-PCR [9] is used to detect TCoV in the intestines of turkey embryos to determine whether or not turkey embryos are infected by TCoV. In this chapter, a protocol for VN assay is described for determining the VN titer of serum from turkeys infected with TCoV or receiving experimental vaccines against TCoV infection. In **step 1**, TCoV stock and serum to be tested are diluted and incubated for neutralization reaction. In **step 2**, the mixture of TCoV and serum is inoculated into embryonated turkey eggs. In **step 3**, the infection of TCoV is determined by the detection of TCoV in the intestines of turkey embryos using IFA assay. In **step 4**, VN titer, the dilution of serum that can inhibit TCoV infection in 50 % of inoculated embryonated turkey eggs, is calculated according to the results of IFA assay [4, 10].

2   Materials

2.1   Neutralization Reaction

1. Turkey coronavirus stock, TCoV/IN/540/94 (GenBank accession number EU022525), is purified through 30–60 % sucrose gradient by ultracentrifugation at $103679 \times g$ for 3 h at 4 °C.

2. Phosphate-buffered saline (PBS) is composed of 1.44 g Na_2HPO_4, 8 g NaCl, 0.24 g KH_2PO_4, and 0.2 g KCl in 1 L ddH_2O. The solution is adjusted to pH 7.2 and autoclaved before use.

2.2   Egg Inoculation

1. Turkey eggs (British United Turkey of America, BUTA) are obtained from Perdue Farm (Washington, IN, USA).

2. Egg incubator (Jamesway, Cambridge, ON, Canada; Natureform, Jacksonville, FL, USA).

3. Egg candling device (Lyon Technologies, Inc. Chula Vista, CA, USA).

2.3   Immunofluorescence Antibody Assay

1. Minotome Plus™ Cryostat (Triangle Biomedical Systems (TBS), Durham, NC, USA).

2. Whirl-Pak bag (Thermo Fisher Scientific, Waltham, MA, USA).

3. Anti-TCoV antiserum to TCoV/IN/540/94.

4. FITC-conjugated goat anti-turkey IgG (H + L) antibody (KPL, Gaithersburg, MD, USA).

5. Vectashield® mounting medium (Vector Laboratories Inc., Burlingame, CA, USA).

6. Fluorescent microscope (Nikon, Melville, NY, USA).

3 Methods

3.1 Neutralization Reaction

3.1.1 TCoV Stock Preparation

1. Inoculate 0.2 mL of TCoV/IN/540/94 into 22-day-old turkey embryos with the procedures identical to those described in Sect. 3.2.

2. Harvest TCoV-containing intestines after 3 days of incubation.

3. Titrate TCoV-containing intestinal homogenate and store at −80 °C freezer (*see* **Note 1**).

3.1.2 Neutralization Reaction

1. Inactivate the serum to be tested at 55 °C in water bath for 30 min.

2. Dilute the serum with sterile PBS in two- or fourfold serially.

3. Take TCoV stock from −80 °C freezer and place the vials directly in a 37 °C water bath for fast thawing process. Right before the virus is completely thawed, remove the vials from the 37 °C water bath and place them on ice (*see* **Note 2**).

4. Dilute TCoV stock to the final concentration of 200 EID_{50}/mL (50 % embryo infectious dose) with sterile PBS.

5. Mix the same volume of the diluted serum and TCoV together and incubate in a 37 °C water bath for 1 h.

3.2 Egg Inoculation

1. Three or five 22-day-old embryonated turkey eggs are used for each dilution of serum to be tested. Each egg is inoculated with 100 µL of diluted serum mixed with 100 µL of 200 EID_{50}/mL TCoV. Embryonated eggs inoculated with serially diluted anti-TCoV serum (with a known titer) mixed with 100 µL of 200 EID_{50}/mL TCoV are used as the positive control for virus neutralization, embryonated eggs inoculated with anti-TCoV serum only are used as the negative control for no virus neutralization, and embryonated eggs inoculated with TCoV only are used as the inoculation control for virus infection.

2. Candle 22-day-old embryonated egg and mark the general location of the embryo at the base of the air cell.

3. Position eggs air cell up and disinfect the area directly at the top of the egg with 70 % ethanol spray. Label eggs.

4. Take eggs to a darkroom because this procedure requires illumination of the egg with an egg candling device while being inoculated.

5. Drill a small hole through the eggshell at the point near the back and head of embryo above the line that separates air cell and the rest of egg.

6. Use a 1 mL syringe with a 22-gauge needle in the length of 1 ½ in. (38 mm) and aim the needle toward the head or back shadow of the embryo. When the end of needle approaches the amniotic sac, give a quick stab toward the embryo to permit the needle to penetrate the amniotic membrane, and then inject 0.2 mL of inoculum (mixture of diluted serum and TCoV). To verify that the needle is in the amniotic sac, carefully move the needle sideways. If the needle has entered the amniotic sac, the embryo should reflect the same movement as the tip of the needle.

7. Seal the holes of eggs with glue and return the eggs to the incubator.

8. Incubate the eggs in the inoculator at 99.3 °F with humidity of 56 % for 3 days until embryonated turkey eggs are 25 days old, 3 days prior to hatching.

3.3 Immunofluorescence Antibody (IFA) Assay

1. After 3 days of incubation, the embryo intestines are harvested.

2. Open the shell via the air cell.

3. Pull the turkey embryo out, and then break the neck quickly.

4. Separate the yolk sac gently.

5. Open the abdominal cavity, and cut the connective tissue between stomach and intestine. Gently separate gall bladder and spleen from intestine.

6. Cut the cloaca and remove the whole intestine from abdomen.

7. Arrange the intestine loop together as a circle and place the intestine in the Whirl-Pak bag (Thermo Fisher Scientific). Snap freeze the intestines in dry ice and store at −80 °C freezer later.

8. Cut frozen intestine sections using the cryotome (TBS Minotome Plus™) and place the sections onto the glass slides.

9. Fix the sections in acetone for 10 min at room temperature (RT).

10. Add 50–100 µL of 2 % goat serum diluted with PBS to each section and incubate at RT for 30 min.

11. Dip slides into ddH$_2$O and wash slides with PBS with stirring for 10 min.

12. Dip slides into ddH$_2$O and get rid of excess water. Leave the slides to air-dry till almost dry.

13. Add 50–100 µL of 1:40 anti-TCoV serum diluted with PBS to each section and incubate at RT for 1 h.

14. Dip slides into ddH$_2$O and wash slides with PBS with stirring for 15 min.

15. Dip slides into ddH$_2$O and get rid of excess water. Leave the slides to air-dry till almost dry.

16. Add 50 to 100 μL of 1:100 FITC-conjugated goat anti-turkey IgG secondary antibody (KPL) diluted with PBS to each section and incubate at RT for 1 h in the dark by covering with aluminum foil or using a covered container.

17. Dip slides into ddH$_2$O and wash slides with PBS with stirring for 15 min.

18. Dip slides into ddH$_2$O and get rid of excess water. Leave the slides to air-dry till almost dry.

19. Place Vectashield® mounting medium (Vector Laboratories) over the sections and cover the slides with cover slips.

20. Observe the green fluorescent signals of TCoV in the intestine for positive IFA on a fluorescent microscope (Nikon). Keep the record of IFA results for further VN titer calculation.

3.4 Calculation of Virus Neutralization (VN) Titer

1. Calculate the number of TCoV-infected or non-infected eggs by IFA results.

2. Calculate the accumulated number of TCoV-infected or non-infected eggs.

3. The VN titer is the dilution of serum that can neutralize TCoV and inhibit TCoV infection in 50 % of embryonated eggs (*see* **Note 3**).

4 Notes

1. Titration of TCoV is to measure the concentration of infectious TCoV in the TCoV-containing intestine homogenate. The infectivity unit of TCoV is the 50 % embryo infectious dose or EID$_{50}$. One EID$_{50}$ unit is the amount of virus that will infect 50 % of virus-inoculated embryonated eggs. Immunofluorescence antibody assay is used to determine the number of turkey embryos infected with TCoV. Example for calculating virus infectivity titer is illustrated below. According to the results of IFA assay, the number of TCoV-infected or non-infected eggs, the accumulated number of TCoV-infected, non-infected, or tested eggs, and the infection percentage of eggs inoculated with tenfold serially diluted TCoV can be calculated (Table 1). The index is calculated by the infection percentage:

Index = [(% Infected at dilution immediately above 50 %) − 50 %]/[(% Infected at dilution immediately above 50 %) − (% Infected at dilution immediately below 50 %)]

% infected at dilution immediately above 50 %: $10^{-3} \rightarrow 62.5$ %

Table 1
Calculation of turkey coronavirus infectivity titer

Dilution	Infected eggs # IFA (+)	Non-infected eggs # IFA (−)	Accumulated # Infected (A)	Non-infected (B)	Tested (A + B)	Infection percentage A/(A + B) × 100 %
10^{-1}	5	0	14	0	14	100 %
10^{-2}	4	1	9	1	10	90 %
10^{-3}	3	2	5	3	8	62.5 %
10^{-4}	2	3	2	6	8	25 %
10^{-5}	0	5	0	11	11	0 %

% infected at dilution immediately below 50 %: $10^{-4} \rightarrow 25$ %
Index $= (62.5$ % $- 50$ %$)/(62.5$ % $- 25$ %$) = 12.5$ %$/37.5$ % $= 0.33$.

The index is then applied to the dilution that produced the percentage infected immediately above 50 %. In this example is the 10^{-3} dilution. The index of 0.33 is applied to this dilution. In this example, the dilution that provided the 50 % infection of eggs or 1 EID_{50} is $10^{-3.33}$.

The reciprocal of this dilution is the amount of virus contained in the 0.2 mL of the original suspension $= 10^{3.33}$ $EID_{50}/0.2$ mL $= 5 \times 10^{3.33}$ $EID_{50}/mL = 1.05 \times 10^4$ EID_{50}/mL. Thus, the infectivity titer of TCoV has been calculated to be 1.05×10^4 EID_{50}/mL.

2. Turkey coronavirus is an enveloped single-stranded RNA virus, so it is very fragile and sensitive to the process of freezing and thawing. It is recommended to use −80 or −20 °C pre-equilibrated CoolBox™ (VWR, Batavia, IL, USA) to transport virus vials from −80 °C freezer to laboratory before dilution and inoculation.

3. Example for calculating VN titer is illustrated below.

   Serum sample A is used for VN titer calculation. Anti-TCoV serum is used as a positive control serum. Both serum A and anti-TCoV serum are diluted into 1:4, 1:16, and 1:64, respectively. Infection of TCoV in the embryonated eggs is determined by IFA assay. The number of TCoV-infected or non-infected eggs, the accumulated number of TCoV-infected, non-infected, or tested eggs, and the infection percentage of eggs inoculated with tenfold serially diluted TCoV can be calculated (Table 2). The index is calculated by the neutralization percentage:
   Index $=$ [(% Neutralized at dilution immediately above 50 %) $-$ 50 %]/[(% Neutralized at dilution immediately above 50 %) $-$ (%Neutralization at dilution immediately below 50 %)].

Table 2
Calculation of turkey coronavirus virus neutralization titer

Titration	Infect # IFA (+)	Non-infect # IFA (−)	Accumulated # Infect (A)	Non-infect (B)	Test (A + B)	Neutralization percentage B/(A + B) × 100 %
NC	0	5	0	5	5	–
TCoV	5	0	5	0	5	0 %
Anti-TCoV serum						
1:4 (4^{-1})	0	5	0	11	11	100 %
1:16 (4^{-2})	1	4	1	6	7	85.7 %
1:64 (4^{-3})	3	2	4	2	6	33.3 %
Serum A						
1:4 (4^{-1})	2	3	2	5	7	71.4 %
1:16 (4^{-2})	3	2	5	2	7	28.6 %
1:64 (4^{-3})	5	0	10	0	10	0 %

1. For anti-TCoV serum, % neutralized at dilution immediately above 50 % is 85.7 % and the dilution is 4^{-2}; % neutralized at dilution immediately below 50 % is 33.3 % and the dilution is 4^{-3}. Therefore, the index is (85.7 % − 50 %)/(85.7 % − 33.3 %) = 0.68.

   The index is then applied to the dilution that produced the percentage neutralized immediately above 50 %, which is 4^{-2} dilution.

   For anti-TCoV serum, the dilution that can provide 50 % neutralization of TCoV on the infection of turkey embryo is $4^{-2.68}$. Therefore, the VN titer of anti-TCoV serum is 1:41.

2. For serum A, % neutralized at dilution immediately above 50 % is 71.4 % and the dilution is 4^{-1}; % neutralized at dilution immediately below 50 % is 28.6 % and the dilution is 4^{-2}. Therefore, the index is (71.4 % − 50 %)/(71.4 % − 28.6 %) = 0.5.

   The index is then applied to the dilution that produced the percentage neutralized immediately above 50 %, which is 4^{-1} dilution.

   For serum A, the dilution that can provide 50 % neutralization of TCoV on the infection of turkey embryo is $4^{-1.5}$. Therefore, the VN titer of anti-TCoV serum is 1:8.

3. In conclusion, anti-TCoV serum has higher VN titer of 1:41 than the VN titer of serum A, which is 1:8.

Acknowledgements

The protocol "Virus neutralization assay for turkey coronavirus infection" illustrated in this chapter had been successfully carried out in the authors' studies on molecular virology, immunology, and/or vaccinology of turkey coronavirus and its related viral enteritis. Those studies had been in part financially supported by USDA, North Carolina Poultry Federation, and/or Indiana Department of Agriculture and technically assisted by Drs. Tom Brien and David Hermes, Mr. Tom Hooper, and Ms. Donna Schrader for clinical serology, virus isolation and propagation, and animal experimentation.

References

1. Loa CC, Lin TL, Wu CC et al (2001) Humoral and cellular immune responses in turkey poults infected with turkey coronavirus. Poult Sci 80:1416–1424

2. Gomaa MH, Yoo D, Ojkic D et al (2008) Seroprevalence of turkey coronavirus in North American turkeys determined by a newly developed enzyme-linked immunosorbent assay based on recombinant antigen. Clin Vaccine Immunol 15:1839–1844

3. Gomaa MH, Yoo D, Ojkic D et al (2009) Use of recombinant S1 spike polypeptide to develop a TCoV-specific antibody ELISA. Vet Microbiol 138:281–288

4. Chen YN, Wu CC, Lin TL (2011) Identification and characterization of a neutralizing-epitope-containing spike protein fragment in turkey coronavirus. Arch Virol 156:1525–1535

5. Loa CC, Lin TL, Wu CC et al (2004) Expression and purification of turkey coronavirus nucleocapsid protein in *Escherichia coli*. J Virol Methods 116:161–167

6. Abdelwahab M, Loa CC, Wu CC et al (2015) Recombinant nucleocapsid protein-based enzyme-linked immunosorbent assay for detection of antibody to turkey coronavirus. J Virol Methods 217:36–41

7. Loa CC, Lin TL, Wu CC et al (2000) Detection of antibody to turkey coronavirus by antibody-capture enzyme-linked immunosorbent assay utilizing infectious bronchitis virus antigen. Avian Dis 44:498–506

8. Nagaraja KV, Pomeroy BS (1980) Immunofluorescent studies on localization of secretory immunoglobulins in the intestines of turkeys recovered from turkey coronaviral enteritis. Am J Vet Res 41:1283–1284

9. Jackwood MW, Boynton TO, Hilt DA et al (2009) Emergence of a group 3 coronavirus through recombination. Virology 398:98–108

10. Thayer SG, Beard CW (2008) Chapter 47: Serologic procedures. In: Dufour-Zavala L, Swayne D, Glisson JR et al (eds) A laboratory manual for the isolation, identification and characterization of avian pathogens, 5th edn. American Association of Avian Pathologist, Athens, GA

Chapter 4

Recombinant Turkey Coronavirus Nucleocapsid Protein Expressed in *Escherichia coli*

Chien Chang Loa, Ching Ching Wu, and Tsang Long Lin

Abstract

Expression and purification of turkey coronavirus (TCoV) nucleocapsid (N) protein from a prokaryotic expression system as histidine-tagged fusion protein are presented in this chapter. Expression of histidine-tagged fusion N protein with a molecular mass of 57 kDa is induced with isopropyl β-D-1-thiogalactopyranoside (IPTG). The expressed N protein inclusion body is extracted and purified by chromatography on nickel-agarose column to near homogeneity. The protein recovery can be 10 mg from 100 ml of bacterial culture. The purified N protein is a superior source of TCoV antigen for antibody-capture ELISA for detection of antibodies to TCoV.

Key words Coronavirus, Nucleocapsid protein, Recombinant protein, Cloning, Protein expression

1 Introduction

Turkey coronavirus (TCoV) is the cause of an acute and highly contagious enteric disease affecting turkeys of all ages. The disease is severe in 1- to 4-week-old turkey poults [1]. Turkey flocks that recover from natural or experimental coronaviral enteritis may develop lifelong immunity [2]. TCoV has been recognized as an important pathogen of young turkeys. TCoV infection causes significant economic losses in the turkey industry due to poor feed conversion and uneven growth. Outbreaks of TCoV enteritis in turkey poults remain as a threat to the turkey industry.

In order to rapidly diagnose and effectively control turkey coronaviral enteritis, development of an antibody-capture enzyme-linked immunosorbent assay (ELISA) for detecting antibodies to TCoV is essential. Development of ELISA for detection of TCoV infection requires large amounts of TCoV antigen. Molecular cloning and expression of TCoV N protein were carried out for preparation of large quantities of highly purified viral proteins.

Coronavirus is an enveloped and positive-stranded RNA virus that possesses three major structural proteins including a

Leyi Wang (ed.), *Animal Coronaviruses*, Springer Protocols Handbooks,
DOI 10.1007/978-1-4939-3414-0_4, © Springer Science+Business Media New York 2016

predominant phosphorylated nucleocapsid (N) protein, peplomeric glycoprotein, and spike (S) protein that makes up the large surface projections of the virion, and membrane protein (M) [3, 4]. The N protein is abundantly produced in coronavirus-infected cells and is highly immunogenic. The N protein binds to the viral genomic RNA and composes the structural feature of helical nucleocapsid.

The N protein is a preferred choice for developing a group-specific serologic assay because of highly conserved sequence and antigenicity. The nucleocapsid proteins of various RNA viruses, such as mumps, rabies, vesicular stomatitis, measles, Newcastle disease, and infectious bronchitis (IBV) viruses, have been used as the coating antigens in diagnostic ELISA [5–10]. Prokaryotic expression is an economic and convenient system to prepare large amount of pure recombinant protein. In addition, the antigenic integrity of N protein expressed in prokaryotic system is expected to be maintained due to the lack of glycosylation. This chapter describes expression and purification of TCoV N protein with a prokaryotic system for preparation of a large quantity of highly purified viral protein, which can be used as coating antigen for antibody-capture ELISA for serologic diagnosis of TCoV infection [11, 12].

2 Materials

2.1 Construction of TCoV N Gene in the Expression Vector pTriEx

1. Virus source (*see* **Note 1**).
2. RNApure reagent (GenHunter, Nashville, TN, USA).
3. Chloroform.
4. Isopropanol.
5. 70 % Ethanol.
6. Diethyl-pyrocarbonate (DEPC)-treated sterile double-distilled water (DEPC-H$_2$O).
7. SuperScript III first-strand synthesis system for RT-PCR kit (Life Technologies/Invitrogen, Carlsbad, CA, USA).
8. RNaseOUT, a recombinant RNase inhibitor (Life Technologies/Invitrogen).
9. RNase H enzyme (Life Technologies/Invitrogen).
10. Random hexamers (Life Technologies/Invitrogen).
11. N gene primers (*see* **Note 2**): NF, 5′-TCTTTTGCCATGGC AAGC-3′; NR, 5′-TTGGGTACCTAAAAGTTCATTCTC-3′.
12. Taq polymerase (Promega Corp, Madison, WI, USA).
13. Pfu polymerase (Stratagene, La Jolla, CA, USA).
14. Deoxynucleotide triphosphates (dNTP) (Promega).
15. Sterile distilled water.

16. pTriEx 1.1 cloning kit (Novagen, Madison, WI, USA; EMD Millipore Corp., Billerica, MA, USA).

17. Vector primer for clone screening: TriExUP primer (Novagen; EMD Millipore Corp.).

18. QIAquick PCR product purification kit (Qiagen, Valencia, CA, USA).

19. Restriction enzymes: Nco I and Kpn I (New England Biolabs, Inc., Ipswich, MA, USA) (*see* **Note 3**).

20. Shrimp alkaline phosphatase (SAP) (Promega Corp).

21. Zymoclean gel DNA recovery kit (Zymo Research, Irvine, CA, USA).

22. *Escherichia coli* (*E. coli*) NovaBlue competent cell (Novagen; EMD Millipore Corp.).

23. Growth medium: LB medium containing 50 µg/ml carbenicillin (Life Technologies, Grand Island, NY, USA).

24. QIAquick mini-prep kit (Qiagen).

25. *E. coli* Tuner (DE3) pLacI competent cell (Novagen; EMD Millipore Corp.).

2.2 Expression of Recombinant TCoV Protein

1. Expression host *E. coli* cell, strain Tuner (DE3) pLacI transformant with recombinant plasmid pTri-N containing N protein gene (prepared from Sects. 2.1 and 3.1).

2. Expression medium: LB medium containing 50 µg/ml carbenicillin, 34 µg/ml chloramphenicol, and 1 % glucose (Life Technologies) (*see* **Note 4**).

3. Isopropyl β-D-1-thiogalactopyranoside (IPTG), 100 mM (Life Technologies).

4. Incubator shaker (New Brunswick Scientific Co., Inc., Edison, NJ, USA; Eppendorf North America, Hauppauge, NY, USA).

2.3 Purification of Recombinant TCoV N Protein

1. BugBuster (Novagen; EMD Millipore Corp.).

2. Benzonase (Novagen; EMD Millipore Corp.).

3. His-Bind column, pre-packed column with 1.25 ml Ni^{2+} charged His-Bind resin (Novagen; EMD Millipore Corp.) (*see* **Note 5**).

4. Binding buffer, 5 mM imidazole, 0.5 M NaCl, 20 mM Tris–HCl (pH 7.9) (Novagen; EMD Millipore Corp.) containing 6 M urea (*see* **Note 6**).

5. Wash buffer, 20 mM imidazole, 0.5 M NaCl, 20 mM Tris–HCl (pH 7.9) (Novagen; EMD Millipore Corp.) containing 6 M urea.

6. Elute buffer, 1 M imidazole, 0.5 M NaCl, 20 mM Tris–HCl (pH 7.9) (Novagen; EMD Millipore Corp.) containing 6 M urea.

7. Protein assay reagent (Bio-Rad, Hercules, CA, USA).

8. SDS-polyacrylamide gel electrophoresis and Western blotting apparatuses (Mini-Protean® electrophoresis chamber and wet/tank blotting system, Bio-Rad).

3   Methods

3.1   Construction of TCoV N Gene in the Expression Vector pTriEx

1. Total RNA was extracted from TCoV virus source by RNApure reagent. Two hundred microliters of virus solution are mixed with 1 ml of RNApure reagent and incubated on ice for 10 min (*see* **Note 7**).

2. Add 180 μl of chloroform, mix the mixture, and vortex vigorously for 10 s (*see* **Note 8**).

3. Centrifuge at $13,000 \times g$ for 10 min at 4 °C. Carefully take the upper aqueous phase into a clean microcentrifuge tube and mix with equal volume of cold isopropanol by vortexing vigorously for 30 s. Incubate on ice for 10 min.

4. Centrifuge at $13,000 \times g$ for 10 min at 4 °C. Carefully discard the supernatant without disturbing the RNA pellet.

5. Wash RNA pellet with 1 ml of cold 70 % ethanol. Incubate on ice for 5 min.

6. Centrifuge at $13,000 \times g$ for 2 min at 4 °C. Remove ethanol. Spin briefly and remove the residual liquid with pipette (*see* **Note 9**).

7. Dissolve RNA pellet in 50 μl of DEPC-H_2O and a portion of it is quantified by spectrophotometry (GeneQuant Pro Spectrophotometer, Amersham Pharmacia Biotech, Inc., Piscataway, NJ, USA; GeneQuant 1300 Spectrophotometer, GE Healthcare Bio-Sciences, Piscataway, NJ, USA) at 260 nm wavelength (*see* **Note 10**).

8. Mix 8 μl (1 pg to 5 μg) of RNA with 1 μl (50 ng/μl) random hexamer and 1 μl (10 mM) dNTP in a total volume of 10 μl.

9. Incubate at 65 °C for 5 min and sit on ice for 1 min.

10. Add 10 μl of SuperScript III cDNA Synthesis Mix (containing 2 μl 10× RT buffer, 4 μl (25 mM) $MgCl_2$, 2 μl (0.1 M) DTT, 1 μl (40 U/μl) RNaseOUT, 1 μl (200 U/μl) SuperScript III RT enzyme) to each RNA/primer mixture.

11. Incubate at 25 °C for 10 min followed by 50 °C for 50 min.

12. Terminate the reverse transcription (RT) reaction at 85 °C for 5 min and chill on ice (*see* **Note 11**).

13. Add 2 μl of the above RT mixture to the PCR amplification reaction (100 μl) with primers NF and NR. A mix of Taq and Pfu at 10:1 is recommended to maintain PCR fidelity (Table 1).

Table 1
Preparation of reaction mixture for turkey coronavirus nucleocapsid protein gene polymerase chain reaction

Components	Volumes (µl)
10× Buffer	10
MgCl$_2$ (25 mM/ml)	6
dNTP (10 mM each)	2
Primer NF (100 ng/µl)	4
Primer NR (100 ng/µl)	4
RT reaction mixture	20
DEPC-H$_2$O	53
Taq/Pfu enzyme	1

14. PCR cyclic parameters: 94 °C for 10 s for denaturation, 58 °C for 30 s for annealing, 72 °C for 2 min for extension for 35 cycles followed by 72 °C for 10-min final extension.

15. PCR product is purified by QIAquick PCR purification kit and recovered in 16 µl of sterile distilled water (pH 7.0–8.5).

16. Add all 16 µl of purified PCR product to the restriction enzyme (RE) digestion with 1 µl (10 units/µl) Nco I, 1 µl (10 units/µl) Kpn I, and 2 µl 10× buffer in one reaction of 20 µl. Incubate at 37 °C for 4 h.

17. Set up the same RE digestion for 1 µg of vector pTriEx 1.1 vector plasmid.

18. For dephosphorylation of digested vector, add 1 µl (1 unit) of SAP to the 20 µl of digestion reaction mixture. Incubate at 37 °C for 30 min.

19. Gel purify both digestion reactions for PCR product and plasmid pTriEx by Zymoclean gel DNA recovery kit. Recover each digested DNA prep in 10 µl of sterile distilled water (*see* **Note 12**).

20. Set up two ligation reactions (pTriEx 1.1 cloning kit) with 1 µl of pTriEx vector and 1 or 4 µl of PCR product (insert) DNA in a reaction of 10 µl as demonstrated in Table 2. Incubate at 16 °C for 15 min (*see* **Note 13**).

21. Take 1 µl of ligation reaction for transformation to NovaBlue competent cell. Plate 20 and 100 µl of the transformation mix on growth medium plates (*see* **Note 14**).

22. Colony screening by PCR with primers TriExUp and NR. The PCR cycling parameters are the same as above for N gene

Table 2
Preparation of ligation reaction mixture for recombinant plasmid carrying turkey coronavirus nucleocapsid protein gene

Components	Volumes (μl)
Vector	x
Insert	y
Sterile water	z
Ligation premix (2×)	5

$(x+y+z=5 \text{ μl})$

amplification (step 14). The PCR product of correct clone is about 1500 bp.

23. The selected clone is grown in growth medium. Plasmids are purified by QIAquick mini-prep kit and sequenced to confirm that the inserted TCoV N gene is in frame with the vector-defined open reading frame at both its N- and C-termini.

24. The recombinant plasmid containing the entire TCoV N protein gene (pTri-N) is transformed to competent *E. coli* strain Tuner (DE3) pLacI. Transformants are grown in expression medium.

3.2 Expression of Recombinant TCoV N Protein

1. A starter culture of expression host bacteria cells is prepared in 3 ml of expression medium. Cells are incubated at 37 °C with shaking at 250 rpm in an incubator shaker overnight, to an OD of 600 nm approximately 0.5 (*see* **Note 15**).

2. The entire 3 ml culture is added to 100 ml of fresh expression medium and incubated at 37 °C with shaking at 250 rpm in an incubator shaker until the OD reached 0.5–1.0 at 600 nm wavelength (*see* **Note 16**).

3. The cultures are induced by addition of IPTG to a final concentration of 1 mM (add 1 ml of sterile 100 mM IPTG solution). The induced cultures are incubated at 37 °C with shaking at 250 rpm in an incubator shaker for another 4 h.

4. The bacterial cultures are harvested by centrifugation at $10,000 \times g$ for 10 min at 4 °C. The cell pellet can be immediately processed or frozen stored at –20 or –80 °C until processed (*see* **Note 17**).

3.3 Purification of Recombinant TCoV N Protein

1. Resuspend the cell pellet completely in 5 ml of BugBuster reagent per gram of wet cell weight (*see* **Note 18**).

2. The nuclease reagent Benzonase is added with 1 μl (25 units) for every ml of BugBuster reagent used.

3. Incubate at room temperature with slow rotation for 20 min.

4. Centrifuge at $16,000 \times g$ for 20 min at 4 °C. The soluble supernatant is discarded and the insoluble fraction (containing inclusion bodies) is dissolved in 10 ml of binding buffer (*see* **Note 19**).

5. Equilibrate His-Bind column with 10 ml of binding buffer. Allow the entire buffer volume to flow through.

6. Apply the protein solution (dissolved inclusion bodies) to the column.

7. Wash the column with 10 ml of binding buffer.

8. Wash the column with 10 ml of wash buffer.

9. Elute the recombinant N protein from the column with 5 ml of elute buffer (*see* **Note 20**).

10. The concentration of purified N protein is determined by protein assay reagent. The yield of purified N protein is about 10 mg from a 100 ml of culture (*see* **Note 21**).

11. The purified N protein is further confirmed by SDS-polyacrylamide gel electrophoresis and Western blotting as a single protein band with a molecular mass of about 57 kDa.

4   Notes

1. Homogenates of infected intestines can be the virus source. For better results, further purification of intestinal homogenates containing TCoV with 40–60 % sucrose gradient is recommended. TCoV/IN/94 (GenBank accession number EU022525) has been used as the stock virus for expression of recombinant TCoV N protein in our laboratory.

2. Primers NF and NR containing restriction sites Nco I and Kpn I, respectively. The amplified product containing the entire open reading frame of TCoV N protein gene (1230 bp).

3. Nco I and Kpn I are typical restriction enzymes. The digestions by both enzymes can be conducted in a single reaction with compatible buffer. For example, the two enzymes from New England Biolabs (Ipswich, MA) can be performed in NE Buffer 1.1.

4. Ampicillin antibiotic marker is on the expression vector pTriEx and chloramphenicol antibiotic marker is on plasmid pLacI in the expression host strain Tuner cells. Carbenicillin is recommended to be in place of ampicillin for better stability for pH changes throughout the bacterial cultures.

5. The binding capacity of 1.25 ml of His-Bind resin is 10 mg of target protein per column. As for any affinity chromatography,

the best purity of target protein is achieved when the amount of protein extract is near the binding capacity.

6. The purpose of 6 M urea is to improve resolution of the sticky inclusion bodies. The presence of 6 M urea does not affect binding of His-Bind resin to target N protein.

7. The suggested ratio of RNApure reagent to sample is 10:1. Excess amount of RNApure reagent has no negative impact. The lower ratio (5:1) in this step is intended to obtain higher concentration of viral RNA in the final supernatants. If the upper aqueous phase after centrifugation at step 3 is more than half of the total volume, there is not enough RNApure reagent added. The appropriate reagent amount may be adjusted. Chloroform is applied at 150 µl for every milliliter of lysate.

8. The sample mixture with chloroform at this step can be stored at −70 °C or even lower temperature before proceeding to the next step.

9. Optional: Inverting the tube for 5–10 min for air-drying of RNA pellet is a helpful tip to completely remove any residual ethanol that may interfere the following RT reaction.

10. It is critical to make sure that the jellylike RNA pellet is completely dissolved into solution by repeat pipetting. The volume (50 µl) of DEPC-H_2O may be adjusted according to RNA pellet size to achieve appropriate concentrations. Concentration can be estimated by taking 1 µl of the RNA solution into 1 ml of water. Read at 260 nm. 1 OD260 = 40 µg. The RNA quality can be further examined by OD 260/280 and 260/230 ratio. The ratio of 260/280 about 2.0 is considered as pure for RNA, while 1.8 is considered pure for DNA. The expected 260/230 ratio is around 2.0–2.2 for pure nucleic acid. If the ratio is appreciably lower, it may indicate the presence of protein, phenol, or other contaminants with strong absorption near 280 or 230 nm. RNA should be stored at −70 °C or even lower temperature.

11. The synthesized cDNA in the RT reaction can be stored at −20 °C or even lower temperature until used.

12. PCR product may be purified. The vector must be gel purified due to the long digested fragment size above 30 bp.

13. The molar ratio between vector and insert is suggested at 1:2 to 1:5. The volumes in this step are illustrated for initial exploration. The concentration of digested vector and insert can be estimated by OD 260 or agarose gel electrophoresis with known amount of DNA of similar size in adjacent wells. The ligation reaction mixture can be stored at 4 °C until used for transformation or at −20 °C for longer term.

14. After plating, the leftover transformation mix can be stored at 4 °C for further plating in the following days at different amount if needed.

15. The starter culture can be prepared from a fresh colony on a plate or directly from a glycerol storage stock. An OD around 0.5 represents a culture at log phase when the cells are at the best condition to expand and for protein expression.

16. This usually takes about 2–3 h to reach the OD range. The higher the OD of starter culture in the previous step, the shorter the time to reach this OD range.

17. The centrifuge tubes should be weighed before and after collection of cell pellet for estimation of wet pellet amount and the volume of BugBuster to be applied in the next step. Frozen storage of cell pellets may improve the extraction efficiency of BugBuster reagents through the freeze/thaw cycle.

18. It is important to completely resuspend the cell pellets for the best results of BugBuster extraction. Higher volume of BugBuster reagent does not have adverse effect. Roughly 10–20 ml of BugBuster reagent should be enough for cell pellets collected from a 100 ml of culture. BugBuster reagent can be added directly to frozen cell pellets. There is no need to wait for the temperature to return to room temperature. Protease inhibitors may be added at this step but usually not necessary.

19. It is critical but somewhat difficult to completely dissolve the sticky inclusion bodies. Repeat pipetting up and down until the protein solution is homogeneous. Any undissolved particles will clot the His-Bind column and affect the purification process. It is advisable to centrifuge the dissolved inclusion body protein solution at $5000–10,000 \times g$ for 10–15 min at 4 °C for clarification before application to the column.

20. Eluate may be collected in fractions such as 0.5 or 1 ml each fraction.

21. The presence of 6 M urea is compatible with the protein assay reagent. The assay range can be adjusted for protein concentrations from low μg/ml to 1 mg/ml with different assay format. The protein concentration of the target N protein eluate as obtained following this process is about 1–2 mg/ml. The presence of 6 M urea has no adverse effect on plate coating for ELISA performance. Given the coating concentration of N protein at 20 μg/ml, the eluate is usually diluted in coating buffer for at least 1:10 to reduce the urea content to less than 600 mM and, subsequently, further diminish any possible effect on ELISA performance. Accordingly, the purified N protein eluate can be directly applied to the ELISA assay for detection of antibodies to TCoV.

Acknowledgements

The protocol "Recombinant turkey coronavirus nucleocapsid protein expressed in *Escherichia coli*" detailed in this chapter had been successfully carried out in the authors' studies on characterization and immunology of turkey coronaviral enteritis. Those studies were in part financially supported by USDA, North Carolina Poultry Federation, and/or Indiana Department of Agriculture and technically assisted by Drs. Tom Brien and David Hermes, Mr. Tom Hooper, and Ms. Donna Schrader for clinical and diagnostic investigation, virus isolation and propagation, and animal experimentation.

References

1. Nagaraja KV, Pomeroy BS (1997) Coronaviral enteritis of turkeys (blue comb disease). In: Calnek BW, Barnes HJ, Beard CW et al (eds) Diseases of poultry, 10th edn. Iowa state University Press, Ames, IA

2. Pomeroy BS, Larsen TC, Deshmukh RD, Patel LB (1975) Immunity to transmissible coronaviral enteritis of turkeys (Blue comb). Am J Vet Res 36:553–555

3. Dea S, Tijssen P (1988) Identification of the structural proteins of turkey enteric coronavirus. Arch Virol 99:173–186

4. Saif LJ (1993) Coronavirus immunogens. Vet Microbiol 37:285–297

5. Linde GA, Granstrom M, Orvell C (1987) Immunoglobulin class and immunoglobulin G subclass enzyme-linked immunosorbent assays compared with microneutralisation assay for sero-diagnosis of mumps infection and determination of immunity. J Clin Microbiol 25:1653–1658

6. Reid-Sanden FL, Sumner JW, Smith JS, Fekadu M, Shaddock JH, Bellini WJ (1990) Rabies diagnostic reagents prepared from a rabies N gene recombinant expressed in baculovirus. J Clin Microbiol 28:858–863

7. Hummel KB, Erdman DD, Heath J, Bellini WJ (1992) Baculovirus expression of the nucleocapsid gene of measles virus and utility of the recombinant protein in diagnostic enzyme immunoassays. J Clin Microbiol 30:2874–2880

8. Ahmad S, Bassiri M, Banerjee AK, Yilma T (1993) Immunological characterization of the VSV nucleocapsid (N) protein expressed by recombinant baculovirus in Spodoptera exigua larva: use in differential diagnosis between vaccinated and infected animals. Virology 192:207–216

9. Errington W, Steward M, Emmerson P (1995) A diagnostic immunoassay for Newcastle disease virus based on the nucleocapsid protein expressed by a recombinant baculovirus. J Virol Methods 55:357–365

10. Ndifuna A, Waters AK, Zhou M, Collisson EW (1998) Recombinant nucleocapsid protein is potentially an inexpensive, effective serodiagnostic reagent for infectious bronchitis virus. J Virol Methods 70:37–44

11. Loa CC, Lin TL, Wu CC, Bryan TA, Hooper T, Schrader D (2004) Expression and purification of turkey coronavirus nucleocapsid protein in *Escheria coli*. J Virol Methods 116:161–167

12. Abdelwahab M, Loa CC, Wu CC, Lin TL (2015) Recombinant nucleocapsid protein-based enzyme-linked immunosorbent assay for detection of antibody to turkey coronavirus. J Virol Methods 217:36–41

Chapter 5

Antibody-Capture Enzyme-Linked Immunosorbent Assay for Detection of Antibody to Turkey Coronavirus Using Infectious Bronchitis Virus or Recombinant Nucleocapsid Protein as Coating Antigen

Chien Chang Loa, Mohamed Abdelwahab, Yi-Ning Chen, Ming-Kun Hsieh, Ching Ching Wu, and Tsang Long Lin

Abstract

Turkey coronavirus (TCoV) infection continues to threaten turkey industry. Because specific treatment and effective vaccination program are not available, rapid and cost-effective detection of antibodies to TCoV infection is an important control measure to monitor the disease status in the fields. Two antibody-capture enzyme-linked immunosorbent assay (ELISA) procedures for detection of antibodies to TCoV are outlined in this chapter. One ELISA method uses chicken infectious bronchitis coronavirus (IBV) as the coating antigen based on antigenic cross-reactivity between TCoV and IBV. The other method relies on a recombinant TCoV nucleocapsid protein. Both methods are useful for serological diagnosis of TCoV infection in the turkey flocks.

Key words Turkey coronavirus, Antibody detection, ELISA, Nucleocapsid, Recombinant protein

1 Introduction

Turkey coronavirus (TCoV) causes an acute and highly contagious enteric disease affecting turkeys of all ages [1, 2]. TCoV is an important pathogen and remains as a serious threat to the turkey industry. There is currently no specific treatment or effective vaccine for TCoV infection. In order to rapidly diagnose and effectively control turkey coronaviral enteritis, serological diagnosis of antibodies to TCoV becomes a critical tool to determine the infectivity of turkeys in the turkey flocks.

Immunofluorescent antibody assay (IFA) for detection of anti-TCoV antibodies has been extensively used for disease outbreaks in the fields. However, IFA procedures are time consuming and labor intensive for handling large numbers of samples. In addition, IFA requires highly trained personnel to prepare frozen sections of

Leyi Wang (ed.), *Animal Coronaviruses*, Springer Protocols Handbooks,
DOI 10.1007/978-1-4939-3414-0_5, © Springer Science+Business Media New York 2016

turkey or turkey embryo intestines and perform fluorescent microscopy.

ELISA method has high specificity and sensitivity and can be applied to large numbers of samples simultaneously. Two ELISA procedures are highlighted in this chapter. One ELISA method utilizing infectious bronchitis virus (IBV) as a coating antigen for detection of antibody to TCoV is based on antigenic cross-reactivity between TCoV and IBV [3]. The other antibody-capture ELISA uses a recombinant TCoV nucleocapsid (N) protein as a coating antigen [4, 5].

Nucleocapsid protein appears to be the most abundant viral polypeptide in coronavirus infected cells during all stages of infection. Nucleocapsid protein is detected from 3 to 5 h after infection, at the same time or earlier than the other structural proteins. The only known posttranslational modification of coronavirus N proteins is phosphorylation [6]. The coronavirus N protein is immunodominant [7]. Subcloning of the TCoV N gene to a prokaryotic expression system has resulted in a high-level induction of recombinant protein in our laboratory [4]. The recombinant TCoV N protein expressed from the prokaryotic system is expected to maintain its antigenic integrity because it is not glycosylated.

2 Materials

2.1 ELISA with IBV as Coating Antigen

1. IBV antibody diagnostic kits from IDEXX (Westbrook, Maine, USA).

2. Positive control (PC) serum is the hyperimmune serum against TCoV (TCoV/IN/540/94) prepared from experimentally infected turkeys.

3. Negative control (NC) serum is collected from 4-month-old normal healthy turkeys grown in the isolation room.

4. Goat anti-turkey IgG (H + L) conjugated with horseradish peroxidase (HRP) (Kirkegaard & Perry Laboratories, Gaithersburg, MD, USA).

5. Blocking buffer: PBS (pH 7.4) + 1 % bovine serum albumin.

6. Wash buffer: PBS (pH 7.4) + 0.05 % Tween 20.

7. Assay buffer: PBS (pH 7.4) + 0.05 % Tween 20 + 1 % bovine serum albumin.

8. Substrate tetramethyl benzidine (TMB) (Sigma-Aldrich Co., St. Louis, MO, USA).

9. Stop solution 2 N HCl acid. (Sigma-Aldrich Co.).

10. Plate reader (Vmax™ model, Molecular Devices Corp., Sunnyvale, CA, USA).

**2.2 ELISA
with Recombinant
TCoV N Protein
as Coating Ag**

1. Recombinant TCoV N protein (refer to Chapter 4).

2. ELISA plate (Nunc MaxiSorp® flat-bottom 96-well plate, eBioscience, Inc., San Diego, CA, USA).

3. Positive control (PC) serum is the hyperimmune serum against TCoV (TCoV/IN/540/94) prepared from experimentally infected turkeys.

4. Negative control (NC) serum is collected from 4-month-old normal healthy turkeys grown in the isolation room.

5. Coating buffer: PBS buffer, pH 7.4.

6. Blocking buffer: PBS (pH 7.4) + 1 % bovine serum albumin.

7. Wash buffer: PBS (pH 7.4) + 0.05 % Tween-20.

8. Assay buffer: PBS (pH 7.4) + 0.05 % Tween-20 + 1 % bovine serum albumin.

9. Goat anti-turkey IgG (H + L) conjugated with HRP (Kirkegaard & Perry Laboratories).

10. Substrate TMB (Sigma-Aldrich Co.).

11. Stop solution 2 N HCl acid (Sigma-Aldrich Co.).

12. Plate reader (Vmax™ model, Molecular Devices Corp.).

3 Methods (*See* Notes 1 and 2)

**3.1 ELISA with IBV
as Coating Antigen**

1. Coating: using commercially available IBV coated plate (*see* **Note 3**).

2. (Optional) Blocking: add 150 μl of Blocking buffer (*see* **Note 4**) to each well. Incubation at 37 °C for 1 h.

3. Samples: wash the plate with Wash buffer for three times. (*see* **Note 7**) Samples including PC and NC are prepared at a minimum required dilution of 1:40 in Assay buffer. The diluted serum samples are added at 100 μl to each corresponding well. Incubation at 37 °C for 1 h (*see* **Note 6**).

4. Conjugate: wash the plate with Wash buffer for five times. Goat anti-turkey IgG (H + L) conjugated with horseradish per-oxidase is diluted at 1:1600 in Assay buffer (*see* **Note 7**) and 100 μl is added to each well. Incubation at 37 °C for 1 h.

5. Substrate: wash the plate with Wash buffer for five times. Add substrate TMB at 100 μl/each well. Incubation in the dark at ambient room temperature for 30 min (*see* **Note 8**).

6. Stop: add 100 μl 2 N HCl to each well.

7. Reading: The absorbance of each well at 450 nm is captured by ELISA plate reader. The ELISA value or S/P ratio of each test serum is calculated as (absorbance value of sample serum minus

absorbance value of negative control serum) divided by (absorbance value of positive control serum minus absorbance value of negative control serum) (*see* **Note 9**).

3.2 ELISA with Recombinant TCoV N Protein as Coating Antigen

1. Coating: Coat the ELISA plates with recombinant TCoV N protein at 20 μg/ml in coating buffer for 100 μl/well (*see* **Note 10**) and incubate at a refrigerator 2–8 °C for 12–16 h (*see* **Note 11**).

2. Blocking: wash the plate with Wash buffer for three times and add 150 μl of Blocking buffer to each well. Incubation at 37 °C for 1 h.

3. Samples: wash the plate with Wash buffer for three times. (*see* **Note 5**) Samples including PC and NC are prepared at a minimum required dilution of 1:800 (*see* **Note 7**) in Assay buffer. The diluted serum samples are added at 100 μl to each corresponding well. Incubation at 37 °C for 1 h (*see* **Note 6**).

4. Conjugate: wash the plate with Wash buffer for five times. Goat anti-turkey IgG (H + L) conjugated with horseradish peroxidase is diluted at 1:10,000 in Assay buffer (*see* **Note 7**) and 100 μl is added to each well. Incubation at 37 °C for 1 h.

5. Substrate: wash the plate with Wash buffer for five times. Add TMB substrate at 100 μl/each well. Incubation in the dark at ambient room temperature for 30 min (*see* **Note 8**).

6. Stop: add 100 μl 2 N HCl to each well.

7. Reading: The absorbance of each well at 450 nm is captured by ELISA plate reader. The ELISA value or S/P ratio of each test serum is calculated as (absorbance value of sample serum minus absorbance value of negative control serum) divided by (absorbance value of positive control serum minus absorbance value of negative control serum) (*see* **Notes 9, 12,** and **13**).

4 Notes

1. Although incubation temperature at 37 °C is described for steps of blocking buffer, samples, and conjugate, incubation at room temperature can be a viable alternative when incubator with temperature control is not conveniently located. Please note that the overall assay reactivity (OD readings) will fluctuate along with daily changes of room temperature. However, the end results of ELISA value (S/P ratio) as normalized by an appropriate positive control analyzed on the same plate will not be affected. It is better to keep a record of room temperature for possible trouble shooting when necessary.

2. In between and in the end of each wash cycle, it is important to tap-dry the plates on a stack of paper towel for lower nonspecific background reactivity.

3. The commercially available ELISA plate coated with a pool of IBV strains including Massachusetts, JMK, Arkansas, Connecticut, Clone 30, D274, and D1466.

4. This blocking step is optional because the commercial dry plate is already blocked through the production process of commercial ELISA kits. The additional blocking step may help rehydrate the coating antigens in the wells before sample incubation step and subsequently enhance assay performance.

5. This wash step may be skipped if preferred. It is okay to add diluted samples after removal of the blocking buffer and tap dry the plate on a stack of paper towels. The presence of blocking buffer residue has limited effect on the next step for sample incubation. The components of blocking buffer including PBS buffer and BSA are also parts of the assay buffer in sample dilutions. This wash step is usually performed in our laboratory to achieve the best possible assay performance.

6. Each sample is analyzed in two wells and the mean ELISA value is reported. When percentage coefficient of variance (%CV) is >20 % and both ELISA values are above cutpoint, the result is not reportable and the sample should be reanalyzed. When one or both of the two values is below cutpoint, the sample is considered negative. Each control samples (HPC, LPC, and NC) are analyzed in duplicate ($N=2$; 4 wells for two reportable values).

7. Pipetting volume below 10 μl may cause inter-assay variation. Any pipetting volume below 5 μl is not recommended. To reduce interday variation of dilutions, two steps of dilution may be considered when necessary such as 1:16 and then 1:100 for a final dilution at 1:1600; 1:20 and then 1:40 for a final dilution at 1:800; 1:100 and then 1:100 for a final dilution at 1:10,000.

8. Color development is a result of HRP enzyme reaction. Laboratory environment such as room temperature may have effect on the reaction rate. It is recommended to check the color development throughout the incubation of 30 min and stop the reaction with acid to prevent overdevelopment or underdevelopment. This may not be easy for the first few runs but not that hard after some experience. It is important to keep the plate from light because the substrate is light sensitive. Wash step may be increased a few more times before the addition of TMB substrate if high background of nonspecific reactivity is observed.

9. Cutoff point determination and system suitability controls: Cutoff point should reflect biological variations among non-infected turkeys in the field in order to differentiate the infected samples with positive results. With IFA remains as the gold

standard for detection of TCoV antibody in the field, it is an appropriate approach to set up cutoff point based on IFA positive and negative populations. Some acceptable approaches are discussed below for considerations.

Logistic regression analysis: ELISA value of serum samples from the field turkey flocks as positive or negative for TCoV by IFA are compared. The cutoff point is calculated from the logistic equation $\ln[P/(1-P)] = \beta 1 X + \beta 0$, where X is the ELISA value. At the optimum cutoff point of the ELISA value, the probability of the sample being negative (P) would be the same as the probability of the sample being positive ($1-P$), i.e., $P = 1 - P = 0.5$ or 50 %. The cutoff point is determined by solving $0 = \beta 1 X + \beta 0$ for X ($\ln[0.5/(1-0.5)] = \ln(1) = 0$). Logistic regression is used to estimate the coefficients $\beta 1$ and $\beta 0$. Statistical computations are performed using SAS program. The sample numbers (N) of IFA positive and negative population should be at least 30.

IFA negative population: ELISA values of serum samples ($N \geq 30$) from the field turkey flocks as negative for TCoV by IFA are populated. Outliers are removed by statistical methods such as Box-plot. Mean and standard deviation (SD) of ELISA values are calculated from the remaining samples. Cutoff point can be calculated for 95 % confidence interval as mean plus 1.645 SD (mean $+ 1.645 \times$ SD) for an estimated 5 % false positive rate.

Normal turkey sera: reactivity of normal turkey sera is consistently at low background signals in both ELISA methods, suggesting analytical variations. Cutoff point based on normal turkey sera does not reflect biological variations and therefore is not functional. ELISA value normalization or cutoff point determination from signals of normal turkey sera is misleading.

Fix OD reading: a fixed OD reading as cutoff point is not appropriate due to normal reading fluctuations between batch runs, between analysts, between days, between laboratories.

Data normalization of raw OD readings with a suitable positive control sample is necessary for appropriate interpretation of unknown samples. Comparison of results from different laboratories is difficult due to the lack of standardized reagents. Data normalization with a standard source of PC may be a helpful factor to narrow down the comparability of results from different laboratories.

For system suitability (batch run acceptance criteria), three controls are recommended in each batch run. Each control is analyzed in duplicate ($N = 2$; total four wells for two reportable values). Positive control serum is prepared in two levels at high positive control (HPC) and low positive control (LPC) and each analyzed in duplicates. Normal turkey serum is analyzed in duplicate as

NC. Wells that contain all reagents except serum samples are non-specific background (blank). The general acceptance criteria for these controls in each batch run are based on OD readings. At least two-thirds of controls should have readings in the following order: $HPC > LPC > NC$.

For data normalization, the reading of LPC is suggested in the calculation of ELISA value or S/P ratio of each test serum.

With a HPC in the calculation of S/P ratio in our laboratory, the optimum cutoff point is 0.18 for antibody-capture ELISA using IBV as the coating antigen, while the optimum cutoff point is 0.2 for ELISA using recombinant TCoV N protein as the coating antigen.

10. Coating buffers of various salts may be applied. Results are comparable with phosphate and carbonate based buffers. There are many different kinds of plates with different performance purpose. MaxiSorp® plate gets consistent results for this ELISA method.

11. Coating overnight is minimum. Coating incubation over the weekend is routinely performed without noticeable impact to the assay. It is generally noted that incubation up to 5 days does not affect the ELISA results.

12. ELISA method with the recombinant TCoV N protein as coating antigen has higher reactivity than that with IBV as coating antigen. The dilution factors for serum samples and conjugates are adjusted accordingly. The minimum required dilution of serum samples is 1:800 for the assay with N protein compared to 1:40 for the assay with the IBV. The conjugate dilution factor is 1:10,000 for the assay with N protein compared to 1:1600 for the assay with the IBV.

13. Prevalence, sensitivity, specificity, predictive values: The assay sensitivity and specificity of both ELISA methods relative to IFA are considered comparable. With assumptions of relative sensitivity at 90 %, relative specificity at 95 %, and disease prevalence at 55 %, positive predictive value (PPV) and negative predictive value (NPV) of these two ELISA methods are estimated below:

$$PPV = \frac{Sensitivity \times prevalence}{Sensitivity \times prevalence + (1 - specificity) \times (1 - prevalence)} = 96\%$$

$$NPV = \frac{Specificity \times (1 - prevalence)}{(1 - sensitivity) \times prevalence + specificity \times (1 - prevalence)} = 89\%$$

Acknowledgements

The protocol "Antibody-capture enzyme-linked immunosorbent assay for detection of antibody to turkey coronavirus using infectious bronchitis virus or recombinant nucleocapsid protein as coating antigen" outlined in this chapter had been successfully carried out in the authors' studies on characterization, immunology, and diagnostic serology of turkey coronavirus infection in turkeys. Those studies were in part financially supported by USDA, North Carolina Poultry Federation, and/or Indiana Department of Agriculture and technically assisted by Drs. Tom Brien and David Hermes, Mr. Tom Hooper, and Ms. Donna Schrader in clinical and diagnostic investigation, virus isolation and propagation, and animal experimentation.

References

1. Nagaraja KV, Pomeroy BS (1997) Coronaviral enteritis of turkeys (blue comb disease). In: Calnek BW, Barnes HJ, Beard CW et al (eds) Diseases of poultry, 10th edn. Iowa State University Press, Ames, IA

2. Pomeroy BS, Larsen TC, Deshmukh RD, Patel LB (1975) Immunity to transmissible coronaviral enteritis of turkeys (Blue comb). Am J Vet Res 36:553–555

3. Loa CC, Lin TL, Wu CC, Bryan AT, Thacker HL, Hooper T, Schrader D (2000) Detection of antibody to turkey coronavirus by antibody-capture enzyme-linked immunosorbent assay utilizing infectious bronchitis virus antigen. Avian Dis 44:498–506

4. Loa CC, Lin TL, Wu CC, Bryan TA, Hooper T, Schrader D (2004) Expression and purification of turkey coronavirus nucleocapsid protein in *Escherichia coli*. J Virol Methods 116: 161–167

5. Abdelwahab M, Loa CC, Wu CC, Lin TL (2015) Recombinant nucleocapsid protein-based enzyme-linked immunosorbent assay for detection of antibody to turkey coronavirus. J Virol Methods 217:36–41

6. Garwes DJ, Bountiff L, Millson GC, Elleman CJ (1984) Defective replication of porcine transmissible gastroenteritis virus in a continuous cell line. Adv Exp Med Biol 173:79–93

7. Ignjatovic J, McWaters GP (1993) Monoclonal antibodies to three structural proteins of avian infectious bronchitis virus: characterization of epitopes and antigenic differentiation of Australian strains. J Gen Virol 72:2915–2922

Part III

Reverse Genetics

Chapter 6

Reverse Genetics of Avian Coronavirus Infectious Bronchitis Virus

Sarah M. Keep, Erica Bickerton, and Paul Britton

Abstract

We have developed a reverse genetics system for the avian coronavirus infectious bronchitis virus (IBV) in which a full-length cDNA corresponding to the IBV genome is inserted into the vaccinia virus genome under the control of a T7 promoter sequence. Vaccinia virus as a vector for the full-length IBV cDNA has the advantage that modifications can be introduced into the IBV cDNA using homologous recombination, a method frequently used to insert and delete sequences from the vaccinia virus genome. Here, we describe the use of transient dominant selection as a method for introducing modifications into the IBV cDNA; that has been successfully used for the substitution of specific nucleotides, deletion of genomic regions, and the exchange of complete genes. Infectious recombinant IBVs are generated in situ following the transfection of vaccinia virus DNA, containing the modified IBV cDNA, into cells infected with a recombinant fowlpox virus expressing T7 DNA dependant RNA polymerase.

Key words Transient dominant selection (TDS), Vaccinia virus, Infectious bronchitis virus (IBV), Coronavirus, Avian, Reverse genetics, Nidovirus, Fowlpox virus, T7 RNA polymerase

1 Introduction

Avian infectious bronchitis virus (IBV) is a gammacoronavirus that is the etiological agent of infectious bronchitis (IB); an acute and high contagious disease of poultry characterized by nasal discharge, snicking, tracheal ciliostasis and rales [1]. IBV replicates primarily in the respiratory tract but also in many other epithelial surfaces including oviducts, enteric surfaces and kidneys [2–5]. Following infection with IBV, egg production and quality may be impaired in layers and weight gain in broilers is reduced [6]. Infected birds are predisposed to secondary bacterial infections such as colibaccilosis and mortality in young chicks is not uncommon. Fecal excretion of the virus is a consequence of replication in the intestinal tract; however, this does not normally result in clinical disease.

Infectious bronchitis was first described in the USA in the 1930s [7–9] and is prevalent in poultry farming across the world due to

Leyi Wang (ed.), *Animal Coronaviruses*, Springer Protocols Handbooks,
DOI 10.1007/978-1-4939-3414-0_6, © Springer Science+Business Media New York 2016

the intensive nature of poultry production, estimated to involve the global production of 55 billion chickens (50 billion broilers and 5 billion layers) on an annual basis. In a report, commissioned by Defra in 2005 [10], IBV was indicated as a major cause of ill health amongst chickens and was implicated as being responsible for more economic loss in the UK poultry industry than any other disease [11, 12]; IBV was estimated to cost the UK economy nearly £19 million per year, mainly due to loss of egg production, with serious implications for animal welfare. The cost of control through vaccination is approximately £5 million per year in the UK.

Coronaviruses are enveloped viruses which replicate in the cell cytoplasm. Coronavirus genomes consist of single stranded positive sense RNA, and are the largest of all the RNA viruses ranging from approximately 27 to 32 kb; the genome of IBV is 27.6 kb. Molecular analysis of the role of individual genes in the pathogenesis of RNA viruses has been advanced by the availability of full-length cDNAs, for the generation of infectious RNA transcripts that can replicate and result in infectious viruses. The assembly of full-length coronavirus cDNAs was hampered due to regions from the replicase gene being unstable in bacteria. We therefore devised a reverse genetics strategy for IBV involving the insertion of a full-length cDNA copy of the IBV genome, under the control of a T7 RNA promoter, into the vaccinia virus genome in place of the thymidine kinase (TK) gene. A hepatitis δ ribozyme (HδR) is located downstream of the coronavirus poly(A) tail followed by a T7 termination sequence. IBV infectious RNA is generated from the T7 promoter immediately adjacent to the 5′ end of the IBV cDNA using T7 RNA polymerase and terminates at the T7 termination sequence downstream of the HδR sequence, which autocleaves itself and the T7-termination sequence at the end of the poly(A) sequence, resulting in an authentic IBV genomic RNA copy. Infectious IBV is recovered in situ in cells both transfected with vaccinia virus DNA and infected with a recombinant fowlpox virus expressing T7 RNA polymerase [13].

One of the main advantages of using vaccinia virus as a vector for IBV cDNA is its ability to accept large quantities of foreign DNA without loss of integrity and stability [14]. A second and equally important advantage is the ability to modify the IBV cDNA within the vaccinia virus vector through transient dominant selection (TDS), a method taking advantage of recombinant events between homologous sequences [15, 16]. The TDS method relies on a three-step procedure. In the first step, the modified IBV cDNA is inserted into a plasmid containing a selective marker under the control of a vaccinia virus promoter. In our case we use a plasmid, pGPTNEB193 (Fig. 1; [17]), which contains a dominant selective marker gene, *Escherichia coli guanine phosphoribosyltransferase* (*Ecogpt*; [18]), under the control of the vaccinia virus P7.5K early/late promoter.

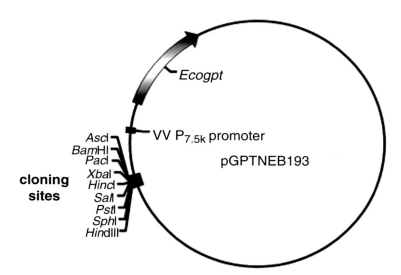

Fig. 1 Schematic diagram of the recombination vector for insertion of genes into a vaccinia virus genome using TDS. Plasmid pGPTNEB193 contains the *Ecogpt* selection gene under the control of the vaccinia virus early/late P$_{7.5K}$ promoter, a multiple cloning region for the insertion of the sequence to be incorporated into the vaccinia virus genome and the *bla* gene (not shown) for ampicillin selection of the plasmid in *E. coli*. For modification of the IBV genome, a sequence corresponding to the region being modified, plus flanking regions of 500–800 nucleotides for recombination purposes is inserted into the multiple cloning sites using an appropriate restriction endonuclease. The plasmid is purified from *E. coli* and transfected into Vero cells previously infected with a recombinant vaccinia virus containing a full-length cDNA copy of the IBV genome

In the second step, this complete plasmid sequence is integrated into the IBV sequence within the vaccinia virus genome (Fig. 2). This occurs as a result of a single crossover event involving homologous recombination between the IBV cDNA in the plasmid and the IBV cDNA sequence in the vaccinia virus genome. The resulting recombinant vaccinia viruses (rVV) are highly unstable due to the presence of duplicate sequences and are only maintained by the selective pressure of the *Ecogpt* gene, which confers resistance to mycophenolic acid (MPA) in the presence of xanthine and hypoxanthine [15]. In the third step, the MPA-resistant rVVs are grown in the absence of MPA selection, resulting in the loss of the *Ecogpt* gene due to a second single homologous recombination event between the duplicated sequences (Fig. 3). During this third step two recombination events can occur; one event will result in the generation of the original (unmodified) IBV sequence and the other in the generation of an IBV cDNA containing the desired modification (i.e., the modification within the plasmid sequence). In theory these two events will occur at equal frequency however in practice this is not necessarily the case.

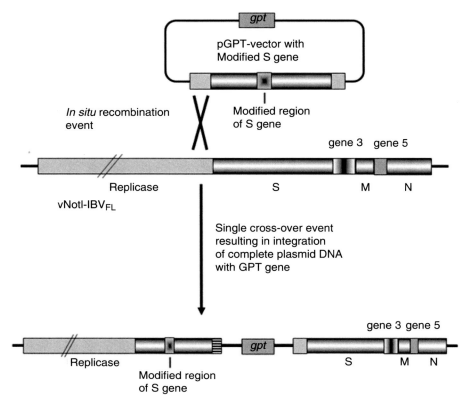

Fig. 2 Schematic diagram demonstrating the TDS method for integrating a modified IBV sequence into the full-length IBV cDNA within the genome of a recombinant vaccinia virus (vNotI-IBVFL). The diagram shows a potential first single-step recombination event between the modified IBV sequence within pGPTNEB193 and the IBV cDNA within vNotI-IBVFL. In order to guarantee a single-step recombination event any potential recombinant vaccinia viruses are selected in the presence of MPA; only vaccinia viruses expressing the *Ecogpt* gene are selected. The main IBV genes are indicated, the replicase, spike (S), membrane (M) and nucleocapsid (N) genes. The IBV gene 3 and 5 gene clusters that express three and two gene products, respectively, are also indicated. In the example shown a modified region of the S gene is being introduced into the IBV genome

To recover infectious rIBVs from the rVV vector, rVV DNA is transfected into primary chick kidney (CK) cells previously infected with a recombinant fowlpox virus expressing T7 RNA polymerase (rFPV-T7; [19]). In addition, a plasmid, pCi-Nuc [13, 20], expressing the IBV nucleoprotein (N), under the control of both the cytomegalovirus (CMV) RNA polymerase II promoter and the T7 RNA promoter, is co-transfected into the CK cells. Expression of T7 RNA polymerase in the presence of the IBV N protein and the rVV DNA, containing the full-length IBV cDNA under the control of a T7 promoter, results in the generation of infectious IBV RNA, which in turn results in the production of infectious rIBVs (Fig. 4). Primary CK cells are refractory for growth of most IBV isolates; therefore rIBVs expressing S glycoproteins from such isolates cannot be recovered using CK cells. In order to recover

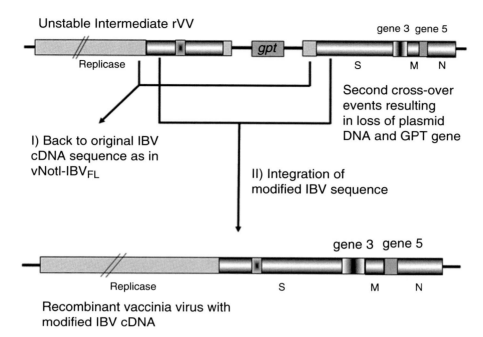

Fig. 3 Schematic diagram demonstrating the second step of the TDS method. Integration of the complete pGPTNEB193 plasmid into the vaccinia virus genome results in an unstable intermediate because of the presence of tandem repeat sequences, in this example the 3′ end of the replicase gene, the S gene and the 5′ end of gene 3. The second single-step recombination event is induced in the absence of MPA; loss of selection allows the unstable intermediate to lose one of the tandem repeat sequences including the *Ecogpt* gene. The second step recombination event can result in either (I) the original sequence of the input vaccinia virus IBV cDNA sequence, in this case shown as a recombination event between the two copies of the 3′ end of the replicase gene which results in loss of the modified S gene sequence along with *Ecogpt* gene; or (II) retention of the modified S gene sequence and loss of the original S gene sequence and *Ecogpt* gene as a result of a potential recombination event between the two copies of the 5′ end of the S gene sequence. This event results in a modified S gene sequence within the IBV cDNA in a recombinant vaccinia virus

such rIBVs, the supernatants from the transfected CK cells are used to infect 10-day-old embryonated hen's eggs. Allantoic fluid is collected and any potential virus passed a further three times in 10-day-old embryos. RNA is extracted from the allantoic fluid of infected eggs and RT-PCR followed by sequencing is used to confirm the identity of the rIBV.

The overall procedure is a multi-step process which can be divided into two parts; the generation of an rVV containing the modified IBV cDNA (Fig. 5) and the recovery of infectious rIBV from the rVV vector (Fig. 4). The generation of the *Ecogpt* plasmids, based on pGPTNEB193, containing the modified IBV cDNA, is by standard *E. coli* cloning methods [21, 22] and is not described here. General methods for growing vaccinia virus have been published by Mackett et al. [23] and for using the TDS method for modifying the vaccinia virus genome by Smith [24].

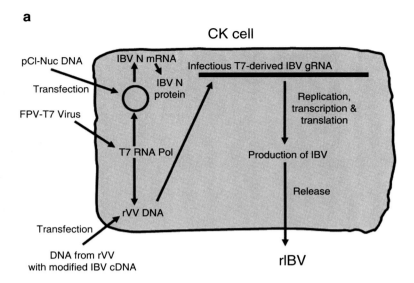

Fig. 4 A schematic representation of the recovery process for obtaining rIBV from DNA isolated from a recombinant vaccinia virus containing a full-length IBV cDNA under the control of a T7 promoter. (a) In addition to the vaccinia virus DNA containing the full-length IBV cDNA under the control of a T7 promoter a plasmid, pCi-Nuc, expressing the IBV nucleoprotein, required for successful rescue of IBV, is transfected into CK cells previously infected with a recombinant fowl pox virus, FPV-T7, expressing T7 RNA polymerase. The T7 RNA polymerase results in the synthesis of an infectious RNA from the vaccinia virus DNA that consequently leads to the generation of infectious IBV being released from the cell. (b) Any recovered rIBV present in the media of P_0 CK cells is used to infect P_1 CK cells. The media is filtered through a 0.22 μm filter to remove any FPV-T7 virus. IBV-induced CPE is normally observed in the P_1 CK cells following a successful recovery experiment. Any rIBV is passaged a further two times, P_2 and P_3, in CK cells. Total RNA is extracted from the P_1 to P_3 CK cells and the IBV-derived RNA analyzed by RT-PCR for the presence of the required modification

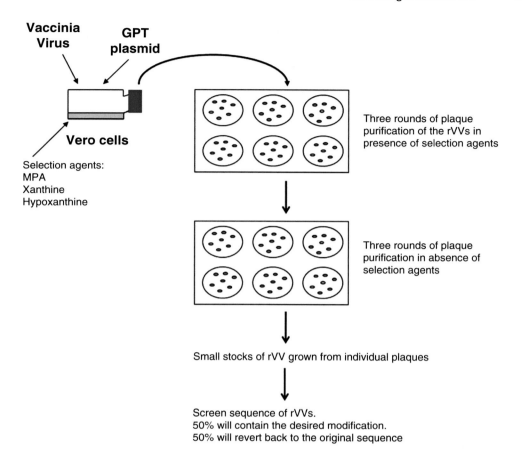

Vaccinia Virus

GPT plasmid

Vero cells

Selection agents:
MPA
Xanthine
Hypoxanthine

Three rounds of plaque purification of the rVVs in presence of selection agents

Three rounds of plaque purification in absence of selection agents

Small stocks of rVV grown from individual plaques

Screen sequence of rVVs.
50% will contain the desired modification.
50% will revert back to the original sequence

Fig. 5 Schematic detailing the multistep process of constructing a recombinant vaccinia virus. Vero cells are infected with rVV containing IBV cDNA and then transfected with a plasmid containing the IBV sequence to be inserted and the selective marker gene *Ecogpt*. Homologous recombination occurs and the complete plasmid sequence is inserted into the rVV. The *Ecogpt* gene allows positive selection of these rVV as it confers resistance to MPA in the presence of xanthine and hypoxanthine. The viruses are plaque purified three times in the presence of selection agents ensuring no wild type VV is present. The removal of the selection agents results in a second recombination event with the loss of the *Ecogpt* gene. Plaque purification in the absence of selection agents not only ensures the loss of the GPT gene but also ensures the maintenance of a single viral population. Small stocks of rVV are grown from individual plaques which are screened through PCR for the desired modification; this is found in theoretically 50 % of rVVs

2   Materials

2.1   Homologous Recombination and Transient Dominant Selection in Vero Cells

1. Vero cells.

2. PBSa: 172 mM NaCl, 3 mM KCl, 10 mM Na_2HPO_4 and 2 mM KH_2PO_4, adjusted to pH 7.2 with HCl.

3. 1× Eagle's Minimum Essential Medium (E-MEM) with Earle's salts, 2 mM L-glutamine, and 2.2 g/l sodium bicarbonate.

4. BES medium: 1× E-MEM, 0.3 % tryptose phosphate broth (TPB), 0.2 % bovine serum albumin (BSA), 20 mM *N,N-Bis*(2-hydroxyethyl)-2-aminoethanesulfonic acid (BES), 0.21 % sodium bicarbonate, 2 mM L-glutamine, 250 U/ml nystatin, 100 U/ml penicillin, and 100 U/ml streptomycin.

5. Opti-MEM 1 with GlutaMAX-1 (Life Technologies).

6. Lipofectin (Life Technologies).

7. Mycophenolic acid (MPA): 10 mg/min 0.1 M NaOH (30 mM); 400× concentrated.

8. Xanthine: 10 mg/ml in 0.1 M NaOH (66 mM); 40× concentrated. Heat at 37 °C to dissolve.

9. Hypoxanthine: 10 mg/ml in 0.1 M NaOH (73 mM); 667× concentrated.

10. Screw-top 1.5 ml microfuge tubes with gasket.

11. Cup form sonicator.

12. 2× E-MEM: 2× E-MEM, 10 % fetal calf serum, 0.35 % sodium bicarbonate, 4 mM L-glutamine, 1000 U/ml nystatin, 200 U/ml penicillin, and 200 U/ml streptomycin.

13. 2 % agar.

14. *Ecogpt* selection medium: 1× E-MEM, 75 μM MPA, 1.65 mM xanthine, 109 μM hypoxanthine, 1 % agar (*see* **Note 1**).

15. Overlay medium: 1× E-MEM, 1 % agar.

16. 1 % Neutral red solution (H_2O).

2.2 Extraction of DNA from Recombinant Vaccinia Virus

1. 20 mg/ml proteinase K.

2. 2× proteinase K buffer: 200 mM Tris–HCl pH 7.5, 10 mM EDTA, 0.4 % SDS, 400 mM NaCl.

3. Phenol–chloroform–isoamyl alcohol (25:24:1).

4. Chloroform.

5. Absolute ethanol.

6. 70 % ethanol.

7. QIAamp DNA mini kit (QIAGEN).

8. 3 M sodium acetate.

2.3 Production of Large Stocks of Vaccinia Virus

1. BHK-21 maintenance medium: Glasgow-Modified Eagle's Medium (G-MEM), 2 mM L-glutamine, 0.275 % sodium bicarbonate, 1 % fetal calf serum, 0.3 % TPB, 500 U/ml nystatin, 100 U/ml penicillin, and 100 U/ml streptomycin.

2. TE buffer: 10 mM Tris–HCl pH 9, 1 mM EDTA.

3. BHK-21 cells.

4. 50 ml Falcon tubes.

2.4 Vaccinia Virus Partial Purification	1. 30 % sucrose (w/v) in 1 mM Tris–HCl pH 9, filtered through 0.22 μm.
	2. Superspin 630 rotor and Sorvall OTD65B ultracentrifuge or equivalent.
2.5 Analysis of Vaccinia Virus DNA by Pulse Field Agarose Gel Electrophoresis	1. 10× TBE buffer: 1 M Tris, 0.9 M boric acid pH 8, and 10 mM EDTA.
	2. Pulsed field certified ultrapure DNA grade agarose.
	3. DNA markers (e.g., 8–48 kb markers, Bio-Rad).
	4. 0.5 mg/ml ethidium bromide.
	5. CHEF-DR® II pulsed field gel electrophoresis (PFGE) apparatus (Bio-Rad) or equivalent.
	6. 6× sample loading buffer: 62.5 % glycerol, 62.5 mM Tris–HCl pH 8, 125 mM EDTA, and 0.06 % bromophenol blue.
2.6 Preparation of rFPV-T7 Stock Virus	1. Chicken embryo fibroblast (CEF) cells.
	2. CEF maintenance medium: 1× 199 Medium with Earle's Salts, 0.3 % TPB, 2 % newborn calf serum (NBCS), 0.225 % sodium bicarbonate, 2 mM L-glutamine, 100 U/ml penicillin, 100 U/ml streptomycin, and 500 U/ml nystatin.
2.7 Recovery of rIBV and Serial Passage on CK Cells	1. Chick kidney (CK) cells.
	2. Stock of rFPV-T7 virus.
	3. The rVV DNA prepared from large partially purified stocks of rVV.
	4. Plasmid pCi-Nuc which contains IBV nucleoprotein under the control of the CMV and T7 promoters.
	5. 0.22 μm syringe driven filters.
	6. 5 ml syringes.

3   Methods

3.1 Infection/ Transfection of Vero Cells with Vaccinia Virus	1. Freeze-thaw the vaccinia virus containing the full-length IBV cDNA genome to be modified three times (37 °C/dry ice) and sonicate for 2 min using a cup form sonicator, continuous pulse at 70 % duty cycle, seven output control (*see* **Notes 2–5**).
	2. Infect 6-well plates of 40 % confluent monolayers of Vero cells with the rVV at a multiplicity of infection (MOI) of 0.2. Use two independent wells per recombination (*see* **Notes 2–5**).
	3. Incubate at 37 °C 5 % CO_2 for 2 h to allow the virus to infect the cells.
	4. After 1 h of incubation, prepare the following solutions for transfection:

Solution A: For each transfection: Dilute 5 μg of modified pGPTNEB193 (containing the modified IBV cDNA) in 1.5 ml of Opti-MEM medium.

Solution B: Dilute 12 μl of Lipofectin in 1.5 ml of Opti-MEM for each transfection.

5. Incubate solutions A and B separately for 30 min at room temperature, then mix the two solutions together and incubate the mixture at room temperature for 15 min.

6. During the 15 min incubation, remove the inoculum from the vaccinia virus infected cells and wash the cells twice with Opti-MEM.

7. Add 3 ml of the transfection mixture (prepared in **step 5**) to each well.

8. Incubate for 60–90 min at 37 °C 5 % CO_2 (*see* **Note 6**).

9. Remove the transfection mixture from each well and replace it with 5 ml of BES medium.

10. Incubate the transfected cells overnight at 37 °C, 5 % CO_2.

11. The following morning add the MXH selection components, MPA 12.5 μl, xanthine 125 μl, and hypoxanthine 7.4 μl, directly to each well (*see* **Note 7**).

12. Incubate the cells at 37 °C 5 % CO_2 until they display extensive vaccinia virus induced cytopathic effect (CPE) (normally 2 days).

13. Harvest the infected/transfected cells into the cell medium of the wells and centrifuge for 3–4 min at $300 \times g$. Discard supernatant and resuspend the pellet in 400 μl 1× E-MEM and store at −20 °C.

3.2 Plaque Purification in the Presence of GPT Selection Agents: Selection of MPA Resistant Recombinant Vaccinia Viruses (GPT+ Phenotype)

1. Freeze-thaw the vaccinia virus produced from Sect. 3.1 three times and sonicate as described in the previous section (Sect. 3.1 **step 1**).

2. Remove the medium from confluent Vero cells in 6-well plates and wash the cells once with PBSa.

3. Prepare 10^{-1} to 10^{-3} serial dilutions of the recombinant vaccinia virus in 1× E-MEM.

4. Remove the PBSa from the Vero cells and add 500 μl of the diluted virus per well.

5. Incubate for 1–2 h at 37 °C 5 % CO_2.

6. Remove the inoculum and add 3 ml of the *Ecogpt* selection medium (*see* **Note 1**).

7. Incubate for 3–4 days at 37 °C 5 % CO_2 and stain the cells by adding 2 ml of 1× E-MEM containing 1 % agar and 0.01 % neutral red.

8. Incubate the cells at 37 °C 5 % CO_2 for 6–24 h and pick 2–3 well isolated plaques for each recombinant, by taking a plug of

agarose directly above the plaque. Place the plug of agar in 400 µl of 1× E-MEM.

9. Perform two further rounds of plaque purification for each selected recombinant vaccinia virus in the presence of *Ecogpt* selection medium, as described in **steps** 1–8 (*see* **Note 8**).

3.3 Plaque Purification in the Absence of GPT Selection Agents: Selection of MPA Sensitive Recombinant Vaccinia Viruses (Loss of GPT+ Phenotype)

1. Take the MPA resistant plaque-purified rVVs which have been plaque purified a total of three times as described in Sect. 3.2 and freeze-thaw and sonicate as described in Sect. 3.1 **step 1**.

2. Remove the medium from confluent Vero cells in 6-well plates and wash the cells with PBSa.

3. Prepare 10^{-1} to 10^{-3} serial dilutions of the recombinant vaccinia virus in 1× E-MEM.

4. Remove the PBSa from the Vero cells and add 500 µl of the diluted virus per well.

5. Incubate for 1–2 h at 37 °C 5 % CO_2.

6. Remove the inoculum and add 3 ml of the overlay medium (*see* **Note 9**).

7. Incubate for 3–4 days at 37 °C 5 % CO_2 and stain the cells by adding 2 ml 1× E-MEM containing 1 % agar and 0.01 % neutral red.

8. Incubate the cells at 37 °C 5 % CO_2 for 6–24 h and pick 3–6 well isolated plaques for each recombinant, by taking a plug of agar directly above the plaque. Place the plug of agar in 400 µl of 1× E-MEM (*see* **Note 8**).

9. Perform two further rounds of plaque purification for each selected recombinant vaccinia virus in the presence of selection medium, as described in **steps** 1–8.

3.4 Production of Small Stocks of Recombinant Vaccinia Viruses

1. Take the MPA sensitive plaque-purified rVVs which have been plaque purified a total of three times as described in Sect. 3.3 and freeze-thaw and sonicate as described in Sect. 3.1 **step 1**.

2. Remove the medium from confluent Vero cells in 6-well plates and wash the cells with PBSa.

3. Dilute 150 µl of the sonicated rVVs in 350 µl of BES medium.

4. Remove the PBSa from the Vero cells and add 500 µl of the diluted rVVs per well.

5. Incubate at 37 °C and 5 % CO_2 for 1–2 h.

6. Add 2.5 ml per well of BES medium.

7. Incubate the infected Vero cells at 37 °C and 5 % CO_2 until the cells show signs of extensive vaccinia virus-induced CPE (approx. 4 days).

8. Scrape the Vero cells into the medium, and harvest into 1.5 ml screw cap tubes with gaskets.

9. Centrifuge for 3 min at $16,000 \times g$ in a benchtop centrifuge.

10. Discard the supernatants and resuspend the cells in a total of 400 µl of BES cell culture medium and store at −20 °C.

3.5   DNA Extraction from Small Stocks of Recombinant Vaccinia Virus for Screening by PCR

There are two methods for DNA extraction:

3.5.1   DNA Extraction Using Phenol–Chloroform–Isoamyl Alcohol

1. To 100 µl of rVV stock produced in Sect. 3.4, add 100 µl 2× proteinase K buffer and 2 µl of the proteinase K stock. Gently mix and incubate at 50 °C for 2 h.

2. Add 200 µl of phenol–chloroform–isoamyl alcohol to the proteinase K-treated samples and mix by inverting the tube 5–10 times and centrifuge at $16,000 \times g$ for 5 min (*see* **Note 10**).

3. Take the upper aqueous phase and repeat step 2 twice more.

4. Add 200 µl of chloroform to the upper phase and mix and centrifuge as in step 2.

5. Take the upper phase and precipitate the vaccinia virus DNA by adding 2.5 volumes of absolute ethanol; the precipitated DNA should be visible. Centrifuge the precipitated DNA at $16,000 \times g$ for 20 min. Discard the supernatant.

6. Wash the pelleted DNA with 400 µl 70 % ethanol and centrifuge at $16,000 \times g$ for 10 min. Discard the supernatant, carefully, and remove the last drops of 70 % ethanol using a capillary tip.

7. Resuspend the DNA in 30 µl water and store at 4 °C (*see* **Note 11**).

3.5.2   Extraction of rVV DNA Using the Qiagen QIAamp DNA Mini Kit

1. Follow the blood/bodily fluids spin protocol and start with 200 µl of rVV stock produced in Sect. 3.4.

2. Elute the rVV DNA in 200 µl buffer AE (provided in the kit) and store at 4 °C.

At this stage the extracted rVV DNA is analyzed by PCR and/or sequence analysis for the presence/absence of the *Ecogpt* gene and for the modifications within the IBV cDNA sequence. Once an rVV is identified that has both lost the *Ecogpt* gene and also contains the desired IBV modification, large stocks are produced. Typically two rVVs will be taken forward at this stage, which ideally have been generated from different wells of the infection/transfection of Vero cells stage previously described in Sect. 3.1. Once the large stocks of the chosen rVVs have been produced, rVV DNA will be extracted and prepared for the recovery of rIBV.

3.6   Production of Large Stocks of Vaccinia Virus

1. Freeze-thaw and sonicate the chosen rVV stocks from Sect. 3.4 as described in Sect. 3.1 **step 1**.

2. Dilute the sonicated virus in BHK-21 maintenance medium and infect $11 \times$ T150 flasks of confluent monolayers of BHK-21

cells using 2 ml of the diluted vaccinia virus per flask at a MOI of 0.1–1.

3. Incubate the infected cells for 1 h at 37 °C and 5 % CO_2.

4. Add 18 ml of pre-warmed (37 °C) BHK-21 maintenance medium and incubate the infected cells at 37 °C and 5 % CO_2 until the cells show an advanced CPE (normally about 2–3 days post-infection). At this stage the cells should easily detach from the plastic.

5. Either continue to step 6 or freeze the flasks in plastic boxes lined with absorbent material and labeled with biohazard tape at –20 °C until further use.

6. If prepared from frozen, the flasks need to be defrosted by leaving them at room temperature for 15 min and then at 37 °C until the medium over the cells has thawed.

7. Tap the flasks to detach the cells from the plastic, if necessary use a cell scraper.

8. Transfer the medium containing the cells to 50 ml Falcon tubes and centrifuge at $750 \times g$ for 15 min at 4 °C to pellet the cells.

9. Discard the supernatant (99 % of vaccinia virus is cell-associated) and resuspend the cells in 1 ml of TE buffer per flask.

10. Pool the resuspended cells then aliquot into screw top microfuge tubes with gasket and store at –70 °C.

11. Use one 1 ml aliquot of the resuspended cells as a virus stock. Use the resuspended cells from the remaining ten flasks for partial purification.

3.7 Vaccinia Virus Partial Purification

1. Freeze-thaw and sonciate the resuspended cells generated from Sect. 3.6 as described in Sect. 3.1 **step 1**.

2. Centrifuge at $750 \times g$ for 10 min at 4 °C to remove the cell nuclei.

3. Keep the supernatant and add TE buffer to give a final volume of 13 ml.

4. Add 16 ml of the 30 % sucrose solution into a Beckman ultraclear (25×89 mm) ultracentrifuge tube and carefully layer 13 ml of the cell lysate from step 3 on to the sucrose cushion.

5. Centrifuge the samples using an ultracentrifuge at $36,000 \times g$, 4 °C for 60 min.

6. The partially purified vaccinia virus particles form a pellet under the sucrose cushion. After centrifugation, carefully remove the top layer (usually pink) and the sucrose layer with a pipette. Wipe the sides of the tube carefully with a tissue to remove any sucrose solution.

7. Resuspend each pellet in 5 ml TE buffer and store at –70 °C.

3.8 Extraction of Vaccinia Virus DNA from Large Partially Purified rVV Stocks

1. Defrost the partially purified vaccinia virus from Sect. 3.7 at 37 °C.

2. Add 5 ml of pre-warmed 2× proteinase K buffer and 100 μl of 20 mg/ml proteinase K to the partially purified vaccinia virus in a 50 ml Falcon tube. Incubate at 50 °C for 2.5 h (*see* **Notes 1–4**).

3. Transfer into a clean 50 ml Falcon tube.

4. Add 5 ml of phenol–chloroform–isoamyl alcohol, mix by inverting the tube 5–10 times, and centrifuge at $1100 \times g$ in a benchtop centrifuge for 15 min at 4 °C. Transfer the upper phase to a clean 50 ml Falcon tube using wide-bore pipette tips (*see* **Notes 10** and **11**).

5. Repeat step 3.

6. Add 5 ml chloroform, mix by inverting the tube 5–10 times, and centrifuge at $1100 \times g$ for 15 min at 4 °C. Transfer the upper phase into a clean 50 ml Falcon tube.

7. Precipitate the vaccinia virus DNA by adding 2.5 volumes of −20 °C absolute ethanol and 0.1 volumes of 3 M sodium acetate. Centrifuge at $1200 \times g$, 4 °C for 60–90 min. A glassy pellet should be visible.

8. Discard the supernatant and wash the DNA using 10 ml −20 °C 70 % ethanol. Leave on ice for 5 min and centrifuge at $1200 \times g$, 4 °C for 30–45 min. Discard the supernatant and remove the last drops of ethanol using a capillary tip. Dry the inside of the tube using a tissue to remove any ethanol.

9. Air-dry the pellet for 5–10 min.

10. Resuspend the vaccinia DNA in 100 μl of water. Do not pipette to resuspend as shearing of the DNA will occur.

11. Leave the tubes at 4 °C overnight. If the pellet has not dissolved totally, add more water.

12. Measure the concentration of the extracted DNA using a NanoDrop or equivalent.

13. Store the vaccinia virus DNA at 4 °C. DO NOT FREEZE (*see* **Note 6**).

3.9 Analysis of Vaccinia Virus DNA by Pulsed Field Agarose Gel Electrophoresis (PFGE)

1. Prepare 2 l of 0.5× TBE buffer for preparation of the agarose gel and as electrophoresis running buffer; 100 ml is required for a 12.7×14 cm agarose gel and the remainder is required as running buffer.

2. Calculate the concentration of agarose that is needed to analyze the range of DNA fragments to be analyzed. Increasing the agarose concentration decreases the DNA mobility within the gel, requiring a longer run time or a higher voltage. However, a higher voltage can increase DNA degradation and reduce resolution. A 0.8 % agarose gel is suitable for separating

DNA ranging between 50 and 95 kb. A 1 % agarose gel is suitable for separating DNA ranging between 20 and 300 kb.

3. Place the required amount of agarose in 100 ml 0.5× TBE buffer and microwave until the agarose is dissolved. Cool to approximately 50–60 °C.

4. Clean the gel frame and comb with MQ water followed by 70 % ethanol. Place the gel frame on a level surface, assemble the comb and pour the cooled agarose into the gel frame. Remove any bubbles using a pipette tip and allow the agarose to set (approx. 30–40 min) and store in the fridge until required.

5. Place the remaining 0.5× TBE buffer into the CHEF-DR® II PFGE electrophoresis tank and switch the cooling unit on. Leave the buffer circulating to cool.

6. Digest 1 μg of the DNA with a suitable restriction enzyme such as Sal I in a 20 μl reaction.

7. Add the sample loading dye to the digested vaccinia virus DNA samples and incubate at 65 °C for 10 min.

8. Place the agarose gel in the electrophoresis chamber; load the samples using wide bore tips and appropriate DNA markers (*see* **Note 11**).

9. The DNA samples are analyzed by PFGE at 14 °C in gels run with a 0.1–1.0 s switch time for 16 h at 6 V/cm at an angle of 120° or with a 3.0–30.0 s switch time for 16 h at 6 V/cm depending on the concentration of agarose used.

10. Following PFGE, place the agarose gel in a sealable container containing 400 ml 0.1 μg/ml ethidium bromide and gently shake for 30 min at room temperature.

11. Wash the ethidium bromide-stained agarose gel in 400 ml MQ water by gently shaking for 30 min.

12. Visualize DNA bands using a suitable UV system for analyzing agarose gels. An example of recombinant vaccinia virus DNA digested with the restriction enzyme *SalI* and analyzed by PFGE is shown in Fig. 6.

3.10 Preparation of rFPV-T7 Stock

Infectious recombinant IBVs are generated in situ by co-transfection of vaccinia virus DNA, containing the modified IBV cDNA, and pCi-Nuc (a plasmid containing the IBV N gene) into CK cells previously infected with a recombinant fowlpox virus expressing the bacteriophage T7 DNA dependant RNA polymerase under the direction of the vaccinia virus P7.5 early–late promoter 8 (rFPV-T7). This protocol covers the procedure for preparing a stock of rFPV/T7 by infecting primary avian chicken embryo fibroblasts (CEFs).

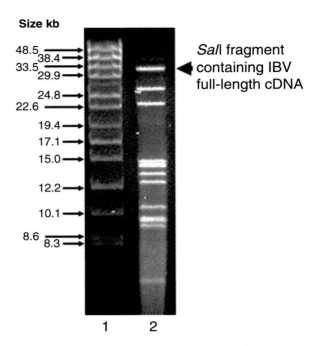

Fig. 6 Analysis of Sal I digested vaccinia virus DNA by PFGE. Lane 1 shows DNA markers and Lane 2 the digested vaccinia virus DNA. The IBV cDNA used does not contain a Sal I restriction site; therefore the largest DNA fragment (~31 kb) generated from the recombinant vaccinia virus DNA represents the IBV cDNA with some vaccinia virus-derived DNA at both ends

Preparation of a 200 ml stock of rFPV-T7 uses ten T150 flasks containing confluent monolayers of CEFs.

1. Remove the culture growth medium from the cells and infect with 2 ml rFPV/T7 at a MOI of 0.1, previously diluted in CEF maintenance medium.

2. Incubate the infected cells for 1 h at 37 °C 5 % CO_2 then without removing the inoculum add 20 ml of CEF maintenance medium.

3. After 4 days post infection check for CPE (90 % of the cells should show CPE). Tap the flasks to detach the cells from the plastic and disperse the cells into the medium by pipetting them up and down.

4. Harvest into 50 ml Falcon tubes and freeze-thaw the cells three times as described in Sect. 3.1 **step 1**.

5. Centrifuge at $750 \times g$, 4 °C for 5 min to remove the cell debris. Take the supernatant containing the virus stock and store at −70 °C until required.

6. Determine the titer of the virus stock using CEF cells. The titer should be in the order of 10^6–10^7 PFU/ml.

3.11 Infection and Transfection of CK Cells for the Recovery of rIBV

1. Wash 40 % confluent CK cells in 6-well plates once with PBSa.

2. Infect the cells with rFPV-T7 at a MOI of 10 in 1 ml of CK cell culture medium. Typically we carry out ten replicates per recovery experiment.

3. Incubate for 1 h at 37 °C 5 % CO_2.

4. During this infection period prepare the transfection reaction solutions.

   Solution A: 1.5 ml Opti-MEM, 10 µg rVV DNA and 5 µg pCi-Nuc per replicate.

   Solution B: 1.5 ml Opti-MEM and 30 µl Lipofectin per replicate.

5. Incubate solutions A and B at room temperature for 30 min.

6. Mix solutions A and B together producing solution AB, and incubate for a further 15 min at room temperature.

7. Remove the rFPV-T7 from each well and wash the CK cells twice with Opti-MEM and carefully add 3 ml of solution AB per well.

8. Incubate the transfected cells at 37 °C 5 % CO_2 for 16–24 h.

9. Remove the transfection medium from each well and replace with 5 ml of BES medium and incubate at 37 °C 5 % CO_2.

10. Two days after changing the transfection media, when FPV/IBV-induced CPE is extensive, harvest the cell supernatant from each well and using a 5 ml syringe, filter through 0.22 µm to remove any rFPV-T7 virus present.

11. Store the filtered supernatant, referred to as passage 0 (P_0CKC) supernatant at −70 °C.

3.12 Serial Passage of rIBVs in CK Cells

To check for the presence of any recovered rIBVs the P_0CKC supernatant is passaged three times, P_1 to P_3, in CK cells (Fig. 4b). At each passage the cells are checked for any IBV-associated CPE and for further confirmation RNA is extracted from P_3 CKC supernatant and is analyzed by RT-PCR (*see* **Note 12**).

For passage 1 (P_1):

1. Wash the confluent CK cells in 6-well plates once with PBSa.

2. Add 1 ml of the P_0CKC supernatant per well and incubate at 37 °C 5 % CO_2 for 1 h.

3. Without removing the inoculum add 2 ml of BES medium per well.

4. Check cells for IBV-associated CPE over the next 2–3 days using a bright-field microscope.

5. Harvest the supernatant from each well and store at −70 °C.

6. Repeat steps 1–6 for passages P_2 and P_3 in CK cells.

7. At P_3 any recovered virus is used to prepare a large stock for analysis of the virus genotype and phenotype.

4 Notes

1. Add an equal volume of 2 % agar to the 2× E-MEM containing MPA, xanthine, and hypoxanthine and mix well before adding it to vaccinia virus infected cells. There is skill to making the overlay medium and adding it to the cells before the agar sets. There are a number of methods including adding hot agar to cold medium, or pre warming the medium to 37 °C and adding agar which has been incubated at 50 °C. Despite the method chosen it is important that all components of the overlay medium are mixed well, and the medium is not too hot when it is added to the cells. If there are problems, 1 % agar can be substituted with 1 % low melting agarose.

2. Vaccinia virus is classified as a category 2 human pathogen and its use is therefore subject to local regulations and rules that have to be followed.

3. Always discard any medium of solution containing vaccinia virus into a 1 % solution of Virkon, leave at least 12 h before discarding.

4. Flasks of cells infected with vaccinia virus should be kept in large plastic boxes, which should be labeled with the word vaccinia and biohazard tape. A paper towel should be put on the bottom of the boxes to absorb any possible spillages.

5. During centrifugation of vaccinia virus infected cells use sealed buckets for the centrifugation to avoid possible spillages.

6. After 2 h of incubation with the transfection mixture, the cells begin to die. It is best therefore not to exceed 90 min incubation.

7. It is important that after the addition of each selection agent, the medium is mixed to ensure the selection agents are evenly distributed. This can be achieved by gently rocking/swirling the plate.

8. The first recombinant event in the TDS system will not necessarily occur in the same place in every rVV. It is therefore important to pick a number of plaques from the first round of plaque purification in presence of GPT selection agents and take a variety of them forward. The following two rounds of plaque purification in the presence of GPT selection agents ensure a single virus population and also that no carry through of the input receiver/wild type vaccinia virus has occurred.

9. Previous chapters and protocols have instructed during plaque purification in the absence of GPT selection agents to plate 10^{-1} rVV dilution in the presence of GPT selection medium and rVV dilutions 10^{-2} and 10^{-3} in the absence. When there are no plaques in the 10^{-1} dilution, it means that the rVV has lost

the GPT gene and the plaques are ready to amplify and check for the presence of mutations.

10. There are risks associated with working with phenol–chloroform–isoamyl alcohol and chloroform. It is important to check the local COSHH guidelines and code of practices.

11. Vaccinia virus DNA is a very large molecule that is very easy to shear, therefore when working with the DNA be gentle and use wide bore tips or cut the ends off ordinary pipette tips. In addition always store vaccinia virus DNA at 4 °C; do not freeze as this leads to degradation. However, there is an exception to this if the vaccinia virus DNA has been extracted using the Qiagen QlAamp DNA mini kit, as this DNA will have already been sheared (the kit only purifies intact DNA fragments up to 50 bp). This DNA can be stored at –20 °C but it is only suitable for analysis of the rVV genome by PCR and is not suitable for the infection and transfection of CK cells for the recovery of rIBV.

12. There is always the possibility that the recovered rIBV is not cytopathic. In this case, check for the presence of viral RNA by RT-PCR at passage 3 (P_3). It is quite common even with a cytopathic rIBV not to see easily definable IBV induced CPE at P_1 and P_2. The recovery process is a low probability event and the serial passage of rIBVs in CK cells acts as an amplification step.

References

1. Britton P, Cavanagh D (2007) Avian coronavirus diseases and infectious bronchitis vaccine development. In: Thiel V (ed) Coronaviruses: molecular and cellular biology. Caister Academic Press, Norfolk, UK

2. Ambali AG, Jones RC (1990) Early pathogenesis in chicks of infection with an enterotropic strain of infectious bronchitis virus. Avian Dis 34:809–817

3. Cavanagh D (2005) Coronaviruses in poultry and other birds. Avian Pathol 34:439–448

4. Cavanagh D, Gelb J Jr (2008) Infectious Bronchitis. In: Saif YM (ed) Diseases of poultry, 12th edn. Blackwell Publishing, Iowa

5. Jones RC (2010) Viral respiratory diseases (ILT, aMPV infections, IB): are they ever under control? Br Poultry Sci 51:1–11

6. Cook JKA, Mockett APA (1995) Epidemiology of infectious bronchitis virus. In: Siddell SG (ed) The coronaviridae. Plenum, New York

7. Schalk AF, Hawn MC (1931) An apparently new respiratory disease of baby chicks. J Am Vet Assoc 78:413–422

8. Beach JR, Schalm OW (1936) A filtrable virus distinct from that of laryngotracheitis: the cause of respiratory disease of chicks. Poult Sci 15:199–206

9. Beaudette FR, Hudson CB (1937) Cultivation of the virus of infectious bronchitis. J Am Vet Med Assoc 90:51–60

10. ZZ0102. Defra report on the Economic assessment of livestock diseases in the United Kingdom (UK) http://randd.defra.gov.uk/Default.aspx?Menu = Menu&Module = More&Location = None&ProjectID = 9781&FromSearch = Y&Publisher = 1&SearchText = ZZ0102&SortString = ProjectCode&SortOrder = Asc&Paging = 10#Description

11. Bennett R (2003) The direct costs of livestock disease: the development of a system of models for the analysis of 30 endemic livestock diseases in Great Britain. J Agric Econ 54:55–71

12. Bennett R, Jpelaar JI (2005) Updated estimates of the costs associated with thirty four endemic livestock diseases in Great Britain. J Agric Econ 56:135–144

13. Casais R, Thiel V, Siddell SG et al (2001) Reverse genetics system for the avian coronavirus infectious bronchitis virus. J Virol 75:12359–12369

14. Thiel V, Siddell SG (2005) Reverse genetics of coronaviruses using vaccinia virus vectors. Curr Top Microbiol Immunol 287:199–227

15. Falkner FG, Moss B (1990) Transient dominant selection of recombinant vaccinia viruses. J Virol 64:3108–3111

16. Britton P, Evans S, Dove B et al (2005) Generation of a recombinant avian coronavirus infectious bronchitis virus using transient dominant selection. J Virol Methods 123:203–211

17. Boulanger D, Green P, Smith T et al (1998) The 131-amino-acid repeat region of the essential 39-kilodalton core protein of fowlpox virus FP9, equivalent to vaccinia virus A4L protein, is nonessential and highly immunogenic. J Virol 72:170–179

18. Mulligan R, Berg P (1981) Selection for animal cells that express the E. coli gene coding for xanthine-guanine phosphoribosyl transferase. Proc Natl Acad Sci U S A 78:2072–2076

19. Britton P, Green P, Kottier S et al (1996) Expression of bacteriophage T7 RNA polymerase in avian and mammalian cells by a recombinant fowlpox virus. J Gen Virol 77:963–967

20. Hiscox JA, Wurm T, Wilson L et al (2001) The coronavirus infectious bronchitis virus nucleoprotein localizes to the nucleolus. J Virol 75:506–512

21. Ausubel FM, Brent R, Kingston RE et al (1987) Current protocols. Molecular biology. Wiley, New York

22. Sambrook J, Fritsch EF, Maniatis T (1989) Molecular cloning: a laboratory manual, 2nd edn. Cold Spring Harbor Laboratory, New York

23. Mackett M, Smith GL, Moss B (1985) The construction and characterisation of vaccinia virus recombinants expressing foreign genes. In: Glover DM (ed) DNA cloning, a practical approach. IRL Press, Oxford, pp 191–211

24. Smith GL (1993) Expression of genes by vaccinia virus vectors. In: Davison MJ, Elliot RM (eds) Molecular virology, a practical approach. IRL Press, Oxford, pp 257–283

Chapter 7

Vaccinia Virus-Based Reverse Genetics for Feline Coronaviruses

Gergely Tekes

Abstract

For decades, the genetic modification of coronavirus genomes and the generation of recombinant corona-viruses have been hampered mostly due to the extraordinary large size of the coronaviral genome. The very first reverse genetic system for feline coronaviruses (FCoVs) was established in the early 2000s; the respective approach exclusively enabled the manipulation of the 3′-third of the viral genome. Later on, vaccinia virus- and bacterial artificial chromosome (BAC)-based systems have been developed. Both systems have the advantage that the entire FCoV genome is amenable for mutagenesis. The main focus of this chapter is the vaccinia virus-based reverse genetic system for FCoVs. Here we present protocols for (1) the generation of a full-length cDNA clone, (2) the manipulation of the FCoV genome, and (3) the rescue of recombinant FCoVs.

Key words Coronavirus, Feline coronavirus (FCoV), Reverse genetics, Infectious clone, Recombinant FCoVs, Vaccinia virus, Homologous recombination, GPT positive selection, GPT negative selection

1 Introduction

The establishment of a reverse genetic system for feline coronaviruses (FCoVs), which allows to modify the entire coronaviral genome, was successfully achieved for the first time in 2008 [1]. This system relies on vaccinia virus, which serves as a cloning vector for the full-length FCoV cDNA. The very first vaccinia virus-based reverse genetic system was developed for the human coronavirus (HCoV) 229 E [2] and since then it has been successfully applied for other coronaviruses, e.g., infectious bronchitis virus (IBV) [3] or mouse hepatitis virus (MHV) [4]. The major advantage of the vaccinia virus-based reverse genetic system lies in the stable integration of full-length corona viral cDNAs into the vaccinia virus genome. In contrast, other conventional cloning techniques often are not suitable for the accommodation of large coronaviral cDNA inserts due to instability of the plasmids caused by certain coronaviral sequences. However, reverse genetic systems,

Leyi Wang (ed.), *Animal Coronaviruses*, Springer Protocols Handbooks,
DOI 10.1007/978-1-4939-3414-0_7, © Springer Science+Business Media New York 2016

which are based on different techniques other than vaccinia virus, have been developed and used successfully for the generation of various recombinant coronaviruses [5–11].

Here, the vaccinia virus-based FCoV reverse genetic system is described. In the first part of this chapter, different strategies for the assembly of the full-length FCoV cDNA and its integration into the vaccinia virus genome are presented (Sect. 3.1). Second, the manipulation of the FCoV cDNA integrated into the vaccinia virus genome is outlined (Sect. 3.2), followed by the recovery of recombinant feline coronaviruses (Sect. 3.3).

2 Materials

2.1 Required for Sect. 3.1

1. Cloning and ligation.

   – pGemT TA cloning kit (Promega).
   – High-concentrated T4 DNA ligase (Fermentas).
   – Antarctic phosphatase (NEB).
   – Qiaex II gel extraction kit (Qiagen).
   – CHEF Mapper-II pulse-field gel electrophoresis System (Bio-Rad).
   – Vaccinia Virus vNotI/tk [12], fowl-pox virus.

2. Vaccinia virus large-scale DNA preparation.

   – BHK-21 cells.
   – DMEM cell culture medium (Sigma).
   – 10× buffer A (10 mM Tris–HCl pH 9.0, 1 mM EDTA).
   – MagNaLyser Green Beads (Roche).
   – MagNaLyser Instrument (Roche).
   – Beckman ultracentrifuge with rotor SW28.
   – Trypsin.
   – RNase-free DNase with the appropriate 10× buffer (Promega).
   – Proteinase K (Roche).
   – 2× proteinase K buffer (200 mM Tris–HCl pH 7.5, 10 mM EDTA pH 8.0, 0.5 % SDS, 400 mM NaCl).
   – RNase-free water.

2.2 Required for Sect. 3.2

1. DMEM cell culture medium (Sigma).
2. CV-1 cells [13].
3. D980R cells [13].

4. Lipofectamine 2000 (Life Technologies).

5. Sonication water bath.

6. Selective medium for GPT positive selection: (1) xanthine (Sigma) 10 mg/ml in 0.1 M NaOH; (2) hypoxanthine (Sigma) 10 mg/ml in 0.1 M NaOH; (3) mycophenolic acid (MPA) (Sigma). For an entire 6-well plate use 12 ml of medium and supplement it with 300 μl xanthine, 18 μl hypoxanthine, and 30 μl MPA from the above described stocks.

7. Selective medium for GPT negative selection: 6-thioguanine (6-TG) (Sigma) 1 mg/ml in 0.1 M NaOH. For an entire 6-well plate use 12 ml of medium and supplement it with 12 μl 6-TG from the above described stock.

2.3   Required for Sect. 3.3

2.3.1   In Vitro RNA Synthesis

1. RiboMax large-scale RNA production system-T7 (Promega).

2. Cap analog 30 mM (7mGpppG) (NEB).

3. RNase inhibitor (Promega).

4. RNase-free DNase (Promega).

5. LiCl solution (7.5 M LiCl, 50 mM EDTA pH 7.5).

6. RNase-free water.

2.3.2   Electroporation

1. Crfk-TetOn-N cells (generated in our laboratory).

2. 1× phosphate-buffered saline (PBS).

3. Electroporator (Bio-Rad Gene Pulser).

4. Electroporation cuvette (4 mm gap) (VWR).

3   Methods

3.1   Integration of the Full-Length FCoV cDNA into the Vaccinia Virus Genome

Two alternative strategies for the assembly of the full-length FCoV infectious clone are described. The first strategy represents a two-step approach (Sect. 3.1.1).This method involves (1) the introduction of the major part of the FCoV genome through in vitro ligation into the vaccinia virus genome (section "Integration of the FCoV cDNA into the Vaccinia Virus Genome via In Vitro Ligation") followed by (2) the completion of the full-length FCoV cDNA via vaccinia virus-mediated homologous recombination (section "Second Step"). The reason for this strategy is that certain coronavirus-derived sequences can cause instability in cloning plasmids, which makes it difficult to assemble the full-length FCoV cDNA by in vitro ligation of FCoV cDNA fragments originating from plasmids. Such an approach was applied for the establishment of the first FCoV infectious clone [1]. Since then, this infectious clone has been successfully applied to study different aspects of FCoV biology [14–16]. In Sect. 3.1.2 an alternative strategy is described, which simplifies the procedure for the generation of the FCoV infectious clone (Tekes, unpublished). This approach omits all of the in vitro ligation steps and it is based exclusively on vaccinia virus-mediated homologous recombination. Regardless of the applied strategy, viral RNA serves as a starting material for the generation of all FCoV-sequence containing plasmids (sections "First Step", 3.1.1.3, "Generation of plasmids suitable for vaccinia virus-mediated homologous recombination").

3.1.1 Two-Step Strategy for the Introduction of the Complete FCoV cDNA into the Vaccinia Virus Genome

First Step

Generation of Plasmids Suitable for the In Vitro Ligation

1. Coronavirus-derived sequences, which can cause instability in cloning vectors, are often located between nt 5000 and 15,000 of the coronaviral genomic sequence. Therefore, this part of the genome should be introduced into the vaccinia virus genome by vaccinia virus-mediated homologous recombination in the second step as described in section "Completion of the FCoV cDNA Using Vaccinia Virus-Mediated Homologous Recombination".

2. Analyze the remaining parts of the FCoV sequence (1–5000 and 15,000–29,000 nt) and choose restriction enzyme sites encoded by the FCoV genome that will allow the in vitro ligation of cloned cDNA inserts. After the analysis, prepare a set of plasmids (no more than 4–5) covering the FCoV genome from nt 1 to 5000 and from nt 15,000 to 29,000 (Fig. 1a).

3. Plasmid A (pA) contains upstream of the FCoV sequence a *Bsp120I* site followed by a T7 promoter and a G nucleotide. The *Bsp120I* site is required for the ligation of the cDNA insert derived from pA with the *NotI* digested vaccinia virus DNA (section "Large-Scale Vaccinia Virus DNA Preparation").The T7 promoter for the T7 RNA polymerase enables the generation of full-length FCoV RNA via in vitro transcription (IVT) (Sect. 3.3.1). The presence of the G nucleotide is recommended for the proper initiation of the T7 polymerase. Furthermore, plasmid D (pD) should contain downstream of the FCoV 3′UTR 20–30 A nucleotides, which will serve as a synthetic poly-A tail after IVT. These A nucleotides should be followed by a unique cleavage site (e.g., *ClaI*), the hepatitis delta ribozyme (HDR) sequence, and a *Bsp120I* cleavage site (Fig. 1a). The digestion of the vaccinia virus DNA with the unique restriction enzyme will enable to terminate the T7 polymerase driven RNA synthesis (Sect. 3.3.1). The HDR sequence fulfills the same function and contributes to the termination of the FCoV RNA. The *Bsp120I* enables the in vitro ligation of the cDNA insert originating from pDinto the *NotI* cleaved vaccinia virus DNA (section "Large-Scale Vaccinia Virus DNA Preparation").

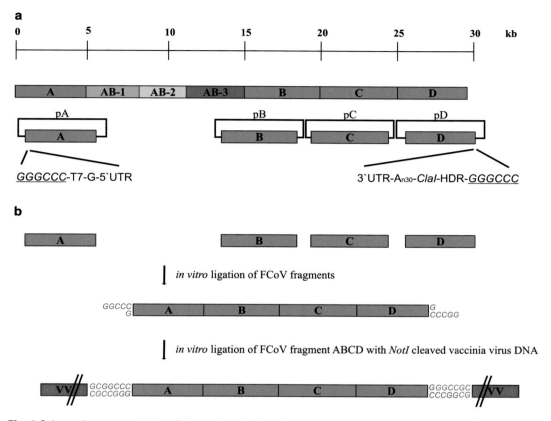

Fig. 1 Schematic representation of the strategy to introduce approximately two-thirds of the FCoV cDNA into the vaccinia virus genome. (a) The nearly 30 kb long FCoV genome, which is divided into seven parts (A, AB-1, AB-2, AB-3, B, C, and D), is depicted. Plasmids A, B, C, and D (pA, pB, pC, and pD) are shown. The detailed descriptions of the 5′ end of fragment A and the 3′ end of fragment D in pA and pD are shown, respectively. In pA the FCoV sequence is preceded by a *Bsp120I* recognition site (*underlined*), T7 DNA-dependent RNA polymerase promoter (T7), and a G nucleotide. In pD the FCoV sequence is followed by poly-A sequence (A_{n30}), *ClaI* cleavage site, hepatitis delta ribozyme (HDR) sequence, and a *Bsp120I* recognition site (*underlined*). (b) Fragments A, B, C, and D (*purple boxes*) derived from plasmids pA, pB, pC, and pD are ligated to obtain fragment ABCD. The overhangs of the *Bsp120I* recognition sites, which enable the ligation into the *NotI* cleaved vaccinia virus DNA, are shown in *purple*. In a further step, fragment ABCD is ligated into the vaccinia virus (VV) genome (*pink boxes*). The overhangs originating from the *NotI* cleavage site in the vaccinia virus DNA and the *Bsp120I* sites from fragment ABCD are depicted in *pink* and *purple*, respectively

In Vitro Ligation of FCoV cDNA Inserts

1. Digest approximately 100 μg of each plasmid with the appropriate restriction enzymes resulting in cDNA fragments A, B, C, and D. In order to avoid the ligation of fragments A and D together through the *Bsp120I* site during the in vitro ligation process (section "In vitro Ligation of FCoV cDNA Inserts"), treat these fragments with alkaline phosphatase. Isolate the fragments using standard gel extraction kit (*see* **Note 1**).

2. Set up an in vitro ligation reaction (total volume 20–30 μl) with all of the fragments in the presence of a high-concentrated T4 DNA ligase overnight at room temperature.

3. Analyze the efficiency of your ligation on an agarose gel after heating up the samples for 5–10 min at 65 °C. If the result of the ligation is not satisfying, repeat the small-scale ligation with different ratios of the fragments. If the desired ligation product can be observed, proceed to the next step.

4. Use the same conditions as in **step 3** for a large-scale ligation. Load the entire reaction on agarose gel and purify the desired ligation product using a gel extraction kit, which enables the efficient recovery of cDNAs larger than 15 kb. For the excision of the band avoid the use of UV-light (*see* **Note 1**). Use this purified product for the ligation with the *NotI* digested vaccinia virus DNA in order to integrate the FCoV cDNA into the vaccinia virus genome (section "Integration of the FCoV cDNA into the Vaccinia Virus Genome via In Vitro Ligation") (Fig. 1b).

Large-Scale Vaccinia Virus DNA Preparation

For the following experiment the vaccinia virus strain *vNotI/tk* is used. This vaccinia virus genome contains only a single *NotI* cleavage site, which enables the introduction of the FCoV cDNA into the vaccinia virus genome via in vitro ligation.

1. Infect four T150 cell culture flasks/dishes of BHK-21 cells (90 % confluent) with vaccinia virus. Harvest the fully infected cells 2–3 days post infection.

2. Pellet the cells at 2000 RPM (4 °C, 3 min).

3. Resuspend the cell pellet in 3 ml of chilled 1× buffer A and fill three MagNaLyser Green Beads with 1 ml suspension each.

4. Homogenize the cells with the MagNaLyser Instrument (Roche) at 5000 RPM for 20 s.

5. Spin the beads for 1–2 min at 2000 RPM (4 °C).

6. Collect the supernatant from the three tubes and combine it into a new tube.

7. Digest the content of the new tube with RNase-free DNase (5U) for 20 min at 37 °C to degrade the remaining cellular DNA in the reaction. Supplement the reaction with the appropriate buffer (10× DNase buffer). Within the virions the vaccinia virus DNA is protected from this digestion step.

8. Inactivate the DNase by adding 20 mM EDTA and incubate the reaction for 20 min at 65 °C.

9. Proceed with trypsin digestion as follows: 0.1 volume of 0.25 % (w/v) trypsin for 20 min at 37 °C.

10. Fill up the reaction volume to 11 ml with chilled 1× buffer A and overlay it on 25 ml 36 % (w/v) sucrose cushion in a 36 ml ultracentrifuge tube. Spin it down for 80 min at 13,500 RPM at 4 °C using a SW 28 rotor.

11. Discard the supernatant and resuspend the pellet in 400 μl buffer A.

12. Add the same volume of 2× proteinase K buffer and 4–5 µl proteinase K to the reaction and incubate for 2 h at 55 °C.

13. After the incubation, pipet 400 µl in two fresh Eppendorf tubes for DNA extraction using phenol–chloroform. Perform the same steps with both reaction tubes (see **Note 2**).

14. Add 400 µl of chilled phenol to the reaction, mix it gently (see **Note 3**) and spin down using a table centrifuge (5 min, 13,000 RPM at 4 °C). Pipet the water phase into a fresh tube and add 400 µl of chilled chloroform. Mix gently and spin again (5 min, 13,000 RPM at 4 °C).

15. Pipet the water phase into a fresh tube and add 1 ml of (2.5 volume) chilled 100 % ethanol to it. Mix carefully and spin down (5 min, 13,000 RPM at 4 °C) (see **Note 2**).

16. Discard the supernatant and wash the DNA pellet with 500–800 µl 70 % ethanol. Spin it down (5 min, 13,000 RPM at 4 °C).

17. Optional: repeat **step 16** to increase the purity of the DNA.

18. Discard the supernatant and add 25 µl of RNase-free water (see **Note 4**).

19. Combine the DNA from both tubes and use everything for the in vitro ligation (see **Note 2**). (section "Integration of the FCoV cDNA into the Vaccinia Virus Genome via In Vitro Ligation").

Integration of the FCoV cDNA into the Vaccinia Virus Genome via In Vitro Ligation

1. Digest the entire amount of the vaccinia virus DNA (from section "Large-Scale Vaccinia Virus DNA Preparation", **step 19**) with *NotI* enzyme for 3–4 h at 37 °C.

2. Add all of the ligated FCoV cDNA insert (from section "In Vitro Ligation of FCoV cDNA Inserts", **step 4**) to the cleaved vaccinia virus DNA and incubate overnight at room temperature in the presence of a high-concentrated DNA ligase and *NotI* restriction enzyme. Supplement the reaction with the appropriate buffers (10× ligation buffer and 10× *NotI* buffer). The volume of the ligation reaction can reach up to 100–150 µl. If necessary, pipet additional *NotI* and/or DNA ligase to the reaction. The presence of *NotI* enzyme prevents the relegation of the vaccinia virus DNA ends.

3. Next day, examine the efficiency of your ligation using pulse field gel electrophoresis (PFGE). Load no more than 5–10 µl aliquot on the gel after heating up the samples for 5–10 min at 65 °C. Freeze the rest of the ligation reaction at −20 °C and use the DNA later for the recovery of vaccinia virus containing the FCoV cDNA (section "Recovery of FCoV cDNA-Containing Vaccinia Virus").

4. If the result of the PFGE is satisfying, proceed with the recovery (see **Note 5**).

*Recovery of FCoV
cDNA-Containing
Vaccinia Virus*

1. Infect almost confluent (90 %) CV-1 cells in one well of a 6-well plate with the fowl-pox virus at an MOI of 5 for 2 h (*see* **Note 6**).

2. Transfect the entire in vitro ligated vaccinia virus DNA (section "Integration of the FCoV cDNA into the Vaccinia Virus Genome via In Vitro Ligation") without further purification using Lipofectamine 2000 (*see* **Note 2**).

3. 5–6 h post transfection: discard the cell culture supernatant, trypsinize, and pellet the cells.

4. Supplement the transfected cells with fresh CV-1 cells (4×10^6) and seed them on a 96-well plate.

5. Incubate the plate at 37 °C until complete cytopathic effect (CPE) develops (5–10 days) in some of the wells.

6. Harvest the cells with CPE and infect fresh CV-1 cells in a well of a 6-well plate with half of the harvested material.

7. Incubate the CV-1 cells until complete CPE develops. Harvest the cells and divide it into two equal aliquots.

8. Take one of the aliquots, pellet the cells and perform vaccinia virus DNA preparation using proteinase K digestion followed by phenol–chloroform extraction as described (section "Large-Scale Vaccinia Virus DNA Preparation", **steps** 12–18).

9. Analyze the presence of the FCoV sequence in the vaccinia virus genome by PCR.

10. If the FCoV sequence was successfully integrated into the vaccinia virus genome, proceed with the second step (section "Generation of Plasmids Suitable for Vaccinia Virus-Mediated Homologous Recombination"). The resulting recombinant vaccinia virus is called vrecFCoV-ABCD.

Second Step

In order to achieve the integration of the full-length FCoV cDNA into the vaccinia virus genome, the remaining part of the FCoV genome (nt 5000–15,000) is introduced by vaccinia virus-mediated homologous recombination.

*Generation of Plasmids
Suitable for Vaccinia
Virus-Mediated
Homologous
Recombination*

1. Generate DNA fragments AB1, AB2, and AB3 by RT-PCR. Clone fragments AB1 and AB3 corresponding approximately to the FCoV sequence nt 4500–8500 and 115,000–15,500, respectively, upstream and downstream of the phosphoribosyl-transferase (GPT) gene in the plasmid pGPT-1 [13] in order to generate pGPT-AB-1/3 (Fig. 2a). The fragment AB-1 contains a 500 nt long overlapping piece at its 5′ terminal with fragment A. Fragment AB-3 possesses a 500 nt long overlapping piece at its 3′ terminal with fragment B. These overlapping sequences are required for the vaccinia virus-mediated homologous recombination. Clone fragment AB2 corresponding approximately to the

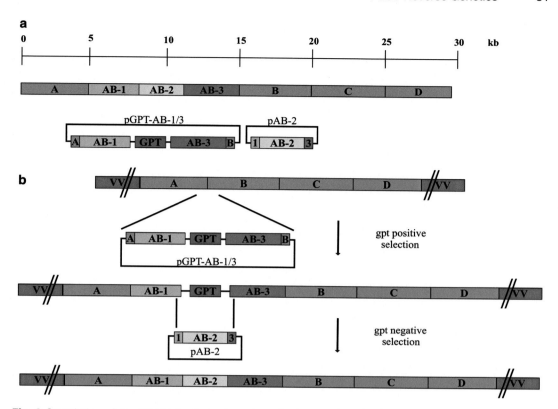

Fig. 2 Completion of the FCoV infectious clone. In order to complete the full-length FCoV cDNA, fragments AB-1, -2, and -3 are introduced using two rounds of vaccinia virus-mediated homologous recombination with GPT positive and GPT negative selection using the plasmids pGPT-AB-1/3 and pAB-2. *GPT* guanine phosphoribosyl transferase

FCoV sequence nt 8000–1200 into a suitable plasmid backbone (Fig. 2a). This fragment contains at both ends 500 nt long overlapping fragments with AB-1 and AB-3, respectively. The overlapping sequences are prerequisites for the vaccinia virus-mediated homologous recombination. The required cleavage sites of AB1, AB2, and AB3 for the cloning reactions must be included through the primer sequences designed for the RT-PCR.

Completion of the FCoV cDNA Using Vaccinia Virus-Mediated Homologous Recombination

The missing part of the FCoV genome (nt 5000–15,000) is introduced by two rounds of vaccinia virus-mediated homologous recombination using GPT as a positive and negative selection marker. The overall strategy is presented in Fig. 2b; the technical details are described in Sect. 3.2.

3.1.2 Alternative Strategy to Generate a Full-Length FCoV Clone Omitting the In Vitro Ligation

If no cloning difficulties are observed with large (4–5 kb) fragments covering the entire FCoV genome, the use of the following method is recommended. One major advantage of this approach is that the time consuming and complicated in vitro ligation steps (sections "In vitro Ligation of FCoV cDNA Inserts" and "Integration of the FCoV cDNA into the Vaccinia Virus Genome via In Vitro Ligation") can be avoided. However, depending on the success of the cloning process, both approaches (Sects. 3.1.1 and 3.1.2) present suitable tools to build an FCoV infectious clone. This alternative strategy involves the introduction of the full-length FCoV cDNA into the vaccinia virus genome using exclusively vaccinia virus-mediated homologous recombination.

Generation of Plasmids Suitable for Vaccinia Virus-Mediated Homologous Recombination

1. Divide the FCoV genome into eight segments. Accordingly, prepare eight fragments by RT-PCR with a size of 3.5–4 kb each covering the entire FCoV genome (Fig. 3).Clone these RT-PCR fragments into a commercial available TA cloning vector in order to generate plasmids 1–8 (p1, p2, p3, p4, p5, p6, p7, and p8).

2. Plasmid 1 (p1) contains upstream of the FCoV sequence a 500 nt long piece of the vaccinia virus genome followed by a T7

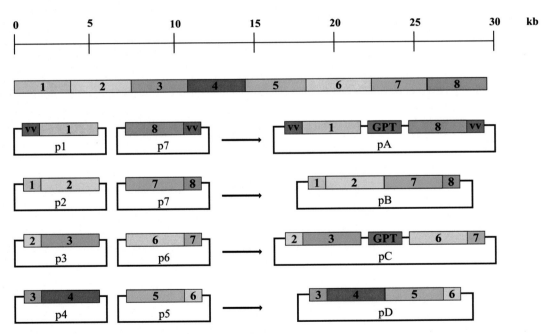

Fig. 3 Generation of plasmids required for the introduction of the full-length FCoV genome into the vaccinia virus genome by vaccinia virus-mediated homologous recombination. For the assembly of the cDNA clone, the approximately 30 kb long FCoV genome is divided into eight overlapping fragments (1–8). The fragments are color-coded. Eight plasmids (p1, p2, p3, p4, p5, p6, p7, and p8) corresponding to these fragments are depicted. Out of these eight plasmids, the generation of four final plasmids (pA, pB, pC, and pD), which are required for the introduction of the entire FCoV cDNA into the vaccinia virus (VV) genome, are shown. The overlapping parts of the various fragments are required for the vaccinia virus-mediated homologous recombination. *GPT* guanosine phosphoribosyl transferase

promoter and a G nucleotide. Plasmid 8 (p8) corresponds to the 3′ end of the FCoV genome sequence followed by 20–30 A nucleotides (synthetic poly-A tail), a unique cleavage site, the hepatitis delta ribozyme (HDR) sequence and a 500 nt long piece of the vaccinia virus genome. Plasmid 2 (p2) contains an approximately 500 nt long overlapping part with p1. Plasmid 7 (p7) has an approximately 500 nt long overlapping part with p8. Plasmid 3 (p3) has an approximately 500 nt long overlapping part with p2. Plasmid 6 (p6) contains an approximately 500 nt long overlapping part with p7. Plasmid 4 (p4) has an approximately 500 nt long overlapping part with p3. Plasmid 5 (p5) comprises an approximately 500 nt long overlapping part with p6. These overlapping parts are required for the vaccinia virus-mediated homologous recombination. In order to finalize the plasmids needed for the vaccinia virus-mediated homologous recombination, additional cloning steps are required (**steps** 3–6).

3. Clone fragments 1 and 8 originating from p1 and p8, respectively, upstream and downstream of the GPT gene in the multiple cloning sites of the pGPT-1. The specific restriction enzyme cleavage sites required for the subcloning originate from the primer sequences used for the generation of the RT-PCR products. The resulting plasmid is called plasmid A (pA) (Fig. 3).

4. Clone fragment 2 originating from p2 in the p7 in order to obtain plasmid B (pB). The specific restriction enzyme cleavage sites required for the subcloning originate from the primer sequences used for the generation of the RT-PCR products.

5. Clone fragments 3 and 6 originating from p3 and p6, respectively, upstream and downstream of the GPT gene in the pGPT-1. The specific restriction enzyme cleavage sites required for the subcloning originate from the primer sequences used for the generation of the RT-PCR products. The resulting plasmid is called plasmid C (pC).

6. Clone fragment 4 originating from p4 in the p5 in order to obtain plasmid D (pD). The cleavage site between fragments 4 and 5 is present in the original FCoV sequence. The other restriction enzyme cleavage sites required for the subcloning originate from the primer sequences used for the generation of the RT-PCR products.

Introduction of the Full-Length FCoV cDNA by Vaccinia Virus-Mediated Homologous Recombination

The entire FCoV genome is introduced by four rounds of vaccinia virus-mediated homologous recombination using GPT as a positive and negative selection marker. The overall strategy is presented in Fig. 4; the technical details are described in Sect. 3.2.

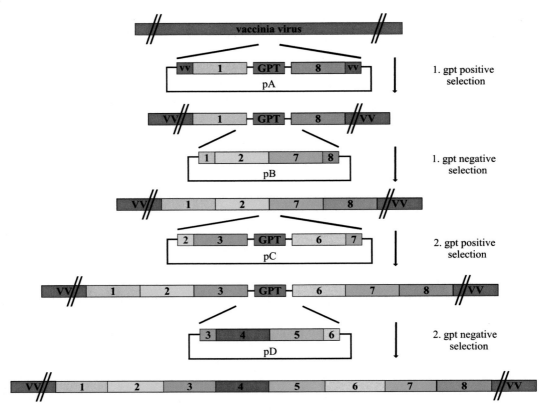

Fig. 4 Strategy for introduction of the full-length FCoV cDNA into the vaccinia virus genome by vaccinia virus-mediated homologous recombination. In order to integrate the full-length FCoV cDNA, fragments 1–8 are introduced via four rounds of vaccinia virus-mediated homologous recombination using GPT as a positive and a negative selection marker. The required plasmids (pA, pB, pC, and pD) and the resulting recombinant vaccinia viruses are shown. *GPT* guanine phosphoribosyl transferase

3.2 Manipulation of the FCoV Genome Vaccinia Virus-Mediated Homologous Recombination

For the manipulation of the FCoV sequence integrated in the vaccinia virus genome, specifically designed plasmids in combination with vaccinia virus-mediated homologous recombination are required. This approach allows the replacement of defined parts of the FCoV genome.

In an initial step, the GPT gene is introduced into the vaccinia virus genome. For this purpose a specific plasmid is required, which contains upstream and downstream of the GPT gene homologous sequences (500 nt) with the targeted FCoV region. These homologous sequences in the plasmid enable the insertion of the GPT gene (preceded by a vaccinia virus promoter) by vaccinia virus-mediated double homologous recombination in the vaccinia virus genome. The resulting recombinant vaccinia virus with GPT gene can be selected using the GPT as a positive selection marker (Sect. 3.2.2).

In the following step, the GPT gene is replaced by the FCoV sequence with the desired mutations. The required specific plasmid contains two homologous regions (500 nt) with the targeted FCoV sequence upstream and downstream of the FCoV sequence to be introduced. Vaccinia virus-mediated homologous recombination leads to replacement of the GPT gene by the FCoV sequence with the desired mutations. In the absence of the GPT gene, the resulting recombinant vaccinia virus can be selected using GPT as a negative selection marker (Sect. 3.2.3).

3.2.1 Infection and Transfection

In order to generate the GPT positive/negative recombinant vaccinia viruses, cells are infected with the appropriate vaccinia virus and transfected with the specifically designed plasmids. During incubation of infected/transfected cells vaccinia virus-mediated homologous recombination takes place between the homologous sequences of the vaccinia genome and the plasmid sequence.

1. Infect CV-1 cells (90 % confluent) in one well of a six-well plate with vaccinia virus (MOI = 1). Incubate the reaction for 2 h at 37 °C.

2. 2 h post infection: transfect the cells with 2–4 µg of the specific plasmid designed for the mutagenesis using Lipofectamine 2000. The transfection is carried out according to the manufacturer's instruction.

3. 5–6 h post transfection: wash the cells and cover them with fresh medium (2 ml).

4. Incubate the infected/transfected cells until complete CPE develops (48–72 h).

5. Harvest the cells by scratching, resuspend in 800 µl of supernatant, and store at −20 °C.

6. This material contains the newly generated GPT positive vs. negative recombinant vaccinia viruses, which will be selected using GPT as positive (Sect. 3.2.2) or negative (Sect. 3.2.3.) selection marker in a following step.

3.2.2 GPT Positive Selection

1. Seed CV-1 cells in a six-well plate 1 day before positive selection starts. On the day of selection the cells should be approximately 90 % confluent.

2. On the next morning, supplement the medium with 25 µg/ml mycophenolic acid (MPA), 250 µg/ml xanthine, and 15 µg/ml hypoxanthine. Incubate the cells for at least 6 h with the GPT positive selection medium.

3. Prepare the vaccinia virus for infection (from Sect. 3.2.1, **step 5**): freeze and thaw the virus three times by placing it into liquid nitrogen followed by sonication (5 min). This step is necessary to release and separate the vaccinia virus particles from the cells.

4. Use 10 µl of different dilutions (stock, 1:10, and 1:100) of this virus for the infection of the CV-1 cells.

5. Incubate the infected cells until single plaques develop (48 h post infection).

6. Pick the plaques (usually six) in 150 µl medium and use 10 µl for the infection of fresh CV-1 cells treated with GPT positive selection medium.

7. Prior infection freeze and thaw the virus as described in **step 3**.

8. Repeat the selection **step 3–4** times.

9. After the last round of selection, infect CV-1 cells in a well of a 6-well plate with 30–40 µl plaque material. Incubate the cells until complete CPE develops (2–4 days). Harvest the cells and divide them into two Eppendorf tubes. One tube should be stored at –20 °C, which can be used later for the GPT negative selection (Sect. 3.2.3). Prepare vaccinia virus DNA from the other half of the reaction to verify the result of the recombination event by PCR.

3.2.3 GPT Negative Selection

1. Seed D980R cells in a six-well plate 1 day before negative selection starts. On the day of selection the cells should be 40 % confluent.

2. On the next morning, supplement the medium with 1 µg/ml 6-thioguanine (6-TG). Incubate the cells at least for 6 h with the GPT negative selection medium.

3. Prepare the vaccinia virus for infection (from Sect. 3.2.2, **step 9**): freeze and thaw the virus three times by placing it into liquid nitrogen followed by sonication (5 min).

4. Use 10 µl of different dilutions (stock, 1:10, and 1:100) of this virus for the infection of the D980R cells.

5. Incubate the infected cells until single plaques develop (48 h post infection).

6. Pick the plaques (usually six) in 150 µl medium and use 10 µl for the infection of fresh D980R cells treated with GPT negative selection medium.

7. Prior infection freeze and thaw the virus as described in **step 3**.

8. Repeat the selection **step 3–4** times.

9. After the last round of selection, infect CV-1 cells in a well of a 6-well plate with 30–40 µl plaque material. Incubate the cells until complete CPE develops (2–4 days). Harvest the cells and divide them into two Eppendorf tubes. One tube should be stored at –20 °C, which can be used later for further mutagenesis. Prepare vaccinia virus DNA from the other half of the reaction to verify the result of the recombination event by PCR.

3.3 Recovery of Recombinant FCoVs

The recovery of recombinant FCoVs comprises the generation of the full-length FCoV RNA by in vitro transcription and the introduction of this RNA into eukaryotic cells. In these cells, the coronaviral life cycle is initiated and the newly produced recombinant viruses are released into the cell culture supernatant.

3.3.1 In Vitro
Transcription (IVT)

Vaccinia virus DNA, which contains the full-length FCoV genome is used as a template for the in vitro transcription.

1. Cells infected with the appropriate vaccinia virus are used for a large-scale DNA preparation as described above (section "Large-Scale Vaccinia Virus DNA Preparation").

2. Digest the entire amount of DNA with a unique cutter restriction enzyme (e.g., *ClaI*) for 3–4 h at 37 °C. The digestion of the vaccinia virus DNA with this enzyme will enable the T7 polymerase driven RNA synthesis to terminate during the in vitro transcription.

3. Perform phenol–chloroform extraction of the digested DNA as described (section "Large-Scale Vaccinia Virus DNA Preparation", **steps** 14–18) and resuspend the DNA pellet in 25 µl RNase-free water (*see* **Note 2**).

4. Used the entire DNA (25 µl) for the in vitro transcription reaction using RiboMaxLarge Scale RNA Production System (Promega). The IVT reaction contains the following components in 50 µl:

3.8 µl	ATP, CTP and UTP (100 mM each)
0.7 µl	GTP (100 mM)
5 µl	Cap Analog (30 mM m7GpppG)
10 µl	5× transcription buffer
5 µl	T7-Enzyme mix
0.5 µl	RNase inhibitor
25 µl	*ClaI* cleaved vaccinia virus DNA

5. Incubate the IVT at 30 °C for 2–3 h.

6. Add 2–4 µl RNase-free DNase to the reaction and incubate for 20 min at 37 °C.

7. Precipitate the RNA using 27 µl LiCl and incubate the reaction at −20 °C for at least 30 min.

8. Spin the reaction (13,000 RPM, 4 °C, 20 min) in order to pellet the RNA.

9. Discard the supernatant and wash the pellet twice with 500 µl 70 % ethanol.

10. Resolve the pellet in 20 µl RNase-free water and analyze 2 µl of it on an agarose gel. This RNA can be stored at −80 °C or directly used for the electroporation (Sect. 3.3.2). However, it is recommended to use the RNA immediately for the electroporation.

3.3.2 Electroporation of the RNA

1. Use for the electroporation an inducible Crfk-Tet/On cell line, which expresses the FCoV N protein.

2. Induce the cells in a 10 cm dish 20–24 h prior electroporation with doxycycline.

3. Trypsinize the cells 20–24 h after induction, pellet (2000 RPM, 4 °C, 3 min) and wash the cells twice with 10 ml of ice cold PBS.

4. Count the cells, pellet again (2000 RPM, 4 °C, 3 min) and resuspend the pellet in PBS to obtain 1×10^6 to 1×10^7 cells in 800 μl.

5. Transfer the 800 μl into a 4 mm gap electroporation cuvette.

6. Add the FCoV RNA (Sect. 3.3.1) to the cells and mix gently.

7. Electroporate the RNA with one pulse using a Gene Pulser II (Bio-Rad) (Resistance: ∞, high-capacity: 950 μF, 0.18 kV) (*see* **Note 7**).

8. Transfer the cells into a 10 cm dish and fill up the dish with 10 ml of fresh medium.

9. Optionally, change the medium 2–3 h after the electroporation.

10. Incubate the cells until CPE develops (usually 2–3 days). Harvest the supernatant containing the recombinant FCoVs and use it for further analysis.

4   Notes

1. Avoid the application of UV-light to excise the bands from the agarose gel. We experienced that exposing the DNA to UV-light can hamper the ligation of these fragments into the vaccinia virus genome. To assess the exact position of a DNA band without damaging it with UV-light, load DNA marker on both sides of your digested fragment on the agarose gel. After electrophoresis, separate the lanes with the marker from the remaining part (contains the digested fragments) of the gel. Using UV-light, cut out a small piece in each of the marker lanes at the expected height of the digested product. Position these lanes back together with the part containing the digested fragment. Cut the agarose gel between the two indicated positions in order to remove the agarose slice with the digested fragment.

2. Do not pipette vaccinia virus DNA with regular tips after proteinase K digestion. These tips can damage the DNA due to their narrow opening. Cut the end of the tips with scissors to enlarge the opening.

3. In order to keep the DNA intact, do not vortex the tubes containing vaccinia virus DNA after proteinase K digestion. Vortexing can break the large vaccinia virus DNA.

4. Do not dry the vaccinia virus pellet but resuspend it immediately in water.

5. In our laboratory CHEF Mapper-II pulse-field gel electrophoresis System (Bio-Rad) is used. For the optimal separation of the bands a 1 % agarose gel should be prepared. The gel runs for approximately 18 h (switch time 3–30 s, angle 120°, voltage 6 V/cm). The set up can vary depending on the system used for PFGE.

6. The vaccinia DNA itself is not infectious. The addition of fowl-pox virus as a helper virus allows the rescue of recombinant vaccinia virus. Furthermore, the infection of CV-1 cells with the fowl-pox virus leads to an abortive infection. After the rescue of the recombinant vaccinia viruses there is no infectious fowl-pox virus present in the reaction.

7. The conditions for the electroporation depend on the cell line and device used for the electroporation. It is recommended to test a given electroporator with the cells to achieve optimal efficiency.

References

1. Tekes G, Hofmann-Lehmann R, Stallkamp I, Thiel V, Thiel HJ (2008) Genome organization and reverse genetic analysis of a type I feline coronavirus. J Virol 82(4):1851–1859. doi:10.1128/JVI.02339-07

2. Thiel V, Herold J, Schelle B, Siddell SG (2001) Infectious RNA transcribed in vitro from a cDNA copy of the human coronavirus genome cloned in vaccinia virus. J Gen Virol 82(Pt 6):1273–1281

3. Casais R, Thiel V, Siddell SG, Cavanagh D, Britton P (2001) Reverse genetics system for the avian coronavirus infectious bronchitis virus. J Virol 75(24):12359–12369. doi:10.1128/JVI.75.24.12359-12369.2001

4. Coley SE, Lavi E, Sawicki SG, Fu L, Schelle B, Karl N, Siddell SG, Thiel V (2005) Recombinant mouse hepatitis virus strain A59 from cloned, full-length cDNA replicates to high titers in vitro and is fully pathogenic in vivo. J Virol 79(5):3097–3106. doi:10.1128/JVI.79.5.3097-3106.2005

5. Almazan F, Gonzalez JM, Penzes Z, Izeta A, Calvo E, Plana-Duran J, Enjuanes L (2000) Engineering the largest RNA virus genome as an infectious bacterial artificial chromosome. Proc Natl Acad Sci U S A 97(10):5516–5521

6. Balint A, Farsang A, Zadori Z, Hornyak A, Dencso L, Almazan F, Enjuanes L, Belak S (2012) Molecular characterization of feline infectious peritonitis virus strain DF-2 and studies of the role of ORF3abc in viral cell tropism. J Virol 86(11):6258–6267. doi:10.1128/JVI.00189-12

7. Almazan F, Dediego ML, Galan C, Escors D, Alvarez E, Ortego J, Sola I, Zuniga S, Alonso S, Moreno JL, Nogales A, Capiscol C, Enjuanes L (2006) Construction of a severe acute respiratory syndrome coronavirus infectious cDNA clone and a replicon to study coronavirus RNA synthesis. J Virol 80(21):10900–10906. doi:10.1128/JVI.00385-06

8. St-Jean JR, Desforges M, Almazan F, Jacomy H, Enjuanes L, Talbot PJ (2006) Recovery of a neurovirulent human coronavirus OC43 from an infectious cDNA clone. J Virol 80(7):3670–3674.doi:10.1128/JVI.80.7.3670-3674.2006

9. Youn S, Leibowitz JL, Collisson EW (2005) In vitro assembled, recombinant infectious bronchitis viruses demonstrate that the 5a open reading frame is not essential for replication. Virology 332(1):206–215. doi:10.1016/j.virol.2004.10.045

10. Yount B, Denison MR, Weiss SR, Baric RS (2002) Systematic assembly of a full-length infectious cDNA of mouse hepatitis virus strain A59. J Virol 76(21):11065–11078

11. Yount B, Curtis KM, Fritz EA, Hensley LE, Jahrling PB, Prentice E, Denison MR, Geisbert TW, Baric RS (2003) Reverse genetics with a full-length infectious cDNA of severe acute respiratory syndrome coronavirus. Proc Natl Acad Sci U S A 100(22):12995–13000. doi:10.1073/pnas.1735582100

12. Merchlinsky M, Moss B (1992) Introduction of foreign DNA into the vaccinia virus genome by in vitro ligation: recombination-independent selectable cloning vectors. Virology 190(1):522–526

13. Hertzig T, Scandella E, Schelle B, Ziebuhr J, Siddell SG, Ludewig B, Thiel V (2004) Rapid identification of coronavirus replicase inhibitors using a selectable replicon RNA. J Gen Virol 85(Pt 6):1717–1725

14. Tekes G, Hofmann-Lehmann R, Bank-Wolf B, Maier R, Thiel HJ, Thiel V (2010) Chimeric feline coronaviruses that encode type II spike protein on type I genetic background display accelerated viral growth and altered receptor usage. J Virol 84(3):1326–1333. doi:10.1128/JVI.01568-09

15. Tekes G, Spies D, Bank-Wolf B, Thiel V, Thiel HJ (2012) A reverse genetics approach to study feline infectious peritonitis. J Virol 86(12):6994–6998. doi:10.1128/JVI.00023-12

16. Thiel V, Thiel HJ, Tekes G (2014) Tackling feline infectious peritonitis via reverse genetics. Bioengineered 5(6):396–400. doi:10.4161/bioe.32133

Part IV

Molecular Diagnostics

Chapter 8

Real-Time RT-PCR Detection of Equine Coronavirus

Fabien Miszczak, Nathalie Kin, Vincent Tesson, and Astrid Vabret

Abstract

Equine coronavirus (ECoV) is a recently identified equine virus, involved mainly in enteric infections. Since the ECoV discovery in 1999, only two real-time RT-PCRs have been developed for viral identification. In this chapter we describe a one-step real-time RT-PCR that has been routinely used in our laboratory for ECoV detection from fecal and respiratory samples.

Key words ECoV, Real-time RT-PCR, Molecular detection, Clinical diagnosis

1 Introduction

Equine coronavirus (ECoV) is a *Betacoronavirus-1* in the lineage A (betacoronavirus A1) that was identified at the end of the last century [1]. ECoV belongs to the genus *Betacoronavirus* and is closely related to human coronavirus OC43 (HCoV-OC43), bovine coronavirus (BCoV), canine respiratory coronavirus (CRCoV), bubaline coronavirus (BuCoV), and porcine hemagglutinating encephalomyelitis virus (PHEV). ECoV was first isolated in North Carolina, USA, from the feces of a diarrheic foal in 1999 (ECoV-NC99) [2]. Multiple ECoV outbreaks have recently been reported in Japan [3, 4] and in the USA [5]. Major clinical signs observed were anorexia, fever, lethargy, leukopenia, and diarrhea, and unspecific discrete symptoms that do not lend to rapid diagnosis. ECoV was mainly detected in fecal samples from horses and less frequently in respiratory secretions [5–7]. A small number of animals with signs of encephalopathic disease have also been observed during these outbreaks [8].

The current diagnosis of ECoV infection can be performed using virus isolation, electron microscopy, serology [9]. A reverse transcription loop-mediated isothermal amplification (RT-LAMP), a non-PCR-based nucleic acid amplification assay, has been recently developed for the detection of ECoV in fecal samples [10]. ECoV was also identified by molecular methods in feces and respiratory samples of foals with and without enteric disease [2, 11, 12]. Real-time RT-PCR assays

Leyi Wang (ed.), *Animal Coronaviruses*, Springer Protocols Handbooks,
DOI 10.1007/978-1-4939-3414-0_8, © Springer Science+Business Media New York 2016

can enable a prompt identification of ECoV in respiratory and fecal samples of horses who were at the early stage of disease onset [5, 6].

2 Materials

2.1 Samples Preparation

2.1.1 Clarification of Fecal Samples

1. Autoclaved 1× Phosphate Buffered Saline (PBS Buffer). For 1 l of 1× PBS buffer, dissolve components as described in Table 1. Dissolve all components in a distillation flask and check pH at 7.4. Then autoclave at 120 °C for 25 min (*see* **Note 1**).

2. pH meter.

3. Autoclave machine or equivalent.

4. Fecal clinical samples stored at +4 °C.

5. 1.5 ml sterile microcentrifuge tubes.

6. Laboratory tabletop centrifuge or equivalent.

2.1.2 Respiratory Samples

1. Respiratory clinical samples stored at −80 °C.

2. Proteinase K Solution (Qiagen®).

3. Heating block or equivalent.

2.2 RNA Extraction

1. QIAsymphony® DSP Virus/Pathogen Mini Kit (Qiagen®).

2. Sample Prep Cartridges, 8-well.

3. 8-Rod Covers.

4. Filter-Tips, 200 and 1500 μl.

5. 2 ml sample tubes, with screw caps and without screw caps, from Sarstedt.

6. ATL buffer (Qiagen®).

7. 300 μl of clinical sample (clarified fecal sample or respiratory sample).

8. QIAsymphony® SP automated instrument (Qiagen®) (*see* **Note 2**).

Table 1
Components for 1 l 1× PBS buffer

Component	Quantity/weight
Autoclaved RNase-free water or its equivalent	1000 ml
Sodium chloride (NaCl) 1.5 M (VWR)	8 g
Potassium chloride (KCl) 30 mM (VWR)	0.2 g
Disodium phosphate (Na_2HPO_4) 80 mM (VWR)	2.9 g
Monopotassium phosphate (KH_2PO_4) 20 mM (BDH Prolabo)	0.2 g

2.3 Real-Time **RT-PCR**	1. Superscript III Platinum One-Step Quantitative RT-PCR System (Invitrogen®).
	2. Superscript® III RT/Platinum Taq® Mix (Invitrogen®).
	3. 10 µM PCR forward primer (ECoV-M-f), 5′-GGTGGAGTT TCAACCCAGAA-3′.
	4. 10 µM PCR reverse primer (ECoV-M-r), 5′-AGGTGCGAC ACCTTAGCAAC-3′.
	5. 10 µM PCR probe (ECoV-M-p), 5′-(6FAM)-CCACAATAAT ACGTGGCCACCTTTA-(BHQ1)-3′ (*see* **Note 3**).
	6. $MgSO_4$ (50 mM) (Invitrogen®).
	7. 2× Reaction Mix (Invitrogen®).
	8. Autoclaved RNase-free water or equivalent.
	9. 0.1 ml strip tubes and caps (Qiagen®).
	10. Loading block (Qiagen®).
	11. Rotor-Gene Q® real-time PCR machine (Qiagen®) (*see* **Note 4**).

3   Methods

The protocol described below is routinely used for ECoV clinical diagnosis in fecal and respiratory samples. Two PCR assays are developed in our laboratory targeting partial M and N genes of the ECoV genome [6]. They were based on short RNA sequences deduced from the ECoV-NC99 strain [13]. The protocol described is based on the highest sensitive PCR targeting the M gene and proved to be a sensitive and useful tool for ECoV detection in field samples (*see* **Note 5**).

3.1 Samples Preparation

3.1.1 Clarification of Fecal Samples

1. Transfer 10–50 % of fecal sample into a 2 ml sterile microcentrifuge tube and adjust to 1 ml with autoclaved 1× PBS buffer.

2. Centrifuge at 3,000 rpm ($850 \times g$) for 30 min at room temperature.

3. Transfer supernatant into a new 1.5 ml sterile microcentrifuge tube.

4. Centrifuge at 10,000 rpm ($9,400 \times g$) for 15 min at room temperature.

5. Collect supernatant and store at +4 °C until RNA extraction.

3.1.2 Respiratory Samples

Respiratory samples (nasopharyngeal swabs) too mucous to be directly extracted with the QIAsymphony® SP automated instrument are previously treated by proteinase K.

1. Add 10 % of proteinase K to the final volume of respiratory specimen in a sterile 2 ml tube.

2. Briefly vortex tubes and incubate at 56 °C for 15 min.

3. Store at +4 °C until RNA extraction.

3.2   RNA Extraction

1. For a new kit, perform the following procedures before samples processing:

   (a) To prepare a carrier RNA stock solution, add 1350 µl buffer AVE to the tube containing 1350 µg lyophilized carrier RNA to obtain a solution of 1 µg/µl. Dissolve the carrier RNA thoroughly and divide it into conveniently sized aliquots. Store the buffer AVE at 2–8 °C for up to 2 weeks.

   (b) Before starting a protocol, check whether precipitate has formed in buffer ATL. If necessary, dissolve by heating at 70 °C with gentle agitation in a water bath and aspirate bubbles from the surface of buffer ATL.

2. Equilibrate all reagents and clinical samples at room temperature before starting the run.

3. Turn on the QIAsymphony® SP automated instrument (Qiagen®).

4. Load the required elution rack into the "Eluate" drawer, and load the required reagent cartridge(s) and consumables into the "Reagents and Consumables" drawer.

5. Perform an inventory scan of the "Reagents and Consumables" drawer.

   Place the samples into the appropriate sample carrier and the tubes containing the carrier RNA–Buffer AVE mixture into the tube carrier.

6. Enter the required information for each batch of samples to be processed:

   (a) Sample information.

   (b) Protocol to be run ("complex200_V6_DSP").

   (c) Elution volume (60 µl) and output position.

   (d) Tubes containing the carrier RNA–Buffer AVE mixture.

7. Run the purification procedure.

8. After the RNA purification, store the purified RNA at 2–8 °C during 24 h before the one-step real-time RT-PCR. For long-term storage of over 24 h, store purified RNA at −20 or −80 °C.

3.3   Real-Time RT-PCR Assay

1. Prepare a one-step RT-PCR master mix sufficient for the designated number of samples in a sterile 1.5 ml microcentrifuge tube on ice, according to Table 2. Include at least one negative control (autoclaved RNase-free water) and one positive control (*see* **Note 6**) for each run. Add additional controls (e.g., purified RNA from the studied samples) as necessary.

2. Insert the strip tubes on the loading block. Aliquot 20 µl of the master mix into separate 0.1 ml strip tubes and label the tubes accordingly.

3. Add 5 μl of each sample and positive control to these tubes. For the negative control, add 5 μl of autoclaved RNase-free water.

4. Close the strip tubes with caps. Insert the strip tubes into the 72-well rotor and lock the rotor into place on the rotor hub of the Rotor-Gene Q® PCR machine.

5. Turn on the real-time PCR machine (Rotor-Gene Q®). Open the "Rotor-Gene Q® series software".

6. Check the "Locking Ring Attached" checkbox and then click "Next".

7. Set the thermal cycle conditions according to Table 3.

8. Run the real-time RT-PCR under the conditions shown.

9. In the "Edit Samples" window, input the necessary information for the corresponding samples (e.g., name of the clinical specimen, positive and negative controls).

Table 2
Components of one-step real-time RT-PCR assay

Reagent	Volume per reaction (μl)	Volume mix for N reactions[a] (μl)	Final concentration
2× Reaction Mix	12.5	$12.5 \times N$	1×
MgSO$_4$ (50 mM)	1.5	$1.5 \times N$	3.0 mM
forward primer (ECoV-M-f) (10 μM)	1.5	$1.5 \times N$	0.6 μM
PCR reverse primer (ECoV-M-r) (10 μM)	1.5	$1.5 \times N$	0.6 μM
PCR probe (ECoV-M-p) (10 μM)	0.5	$0.5 \times N$	0.2 μM
Superscript® III RT/Platinum Taq® Mix	0.5	$0.5 \times N$	–
Autoclaved RNase-free water or equivalent	2	$2 \times N$	–
Total	20	$20 \times N$	–

[a] N = number of 0.1 ml strip tubes

Table 3
Conditions for the one-step real-time RT-PCR assay

Step	Temperature (°C)	Time
1. Reverse transcription	50	15 min
2. Initial PCR activation step	95	2 min
3. Thermal cycling (45 cycles)		
Denaturation	95	15 s
Annealing and extension	60	60 s

10. After performing the RT-PCR, examine the amplification curves of the reactions and the corresponding threshold cycles (Ct). Positive clinical samples will generate amplification curves above the threshold line, and negative samples and water control will be, by contrast, below the threshold line (Fig. 1a). Based on the Ct values from tenfold serial dilutions of a reference standard, the RT-PCR can be used to quantify the amount of input target in the positive samples by comparison with the reference (Fig. 1b). This amount can be automatically calculated by the software.

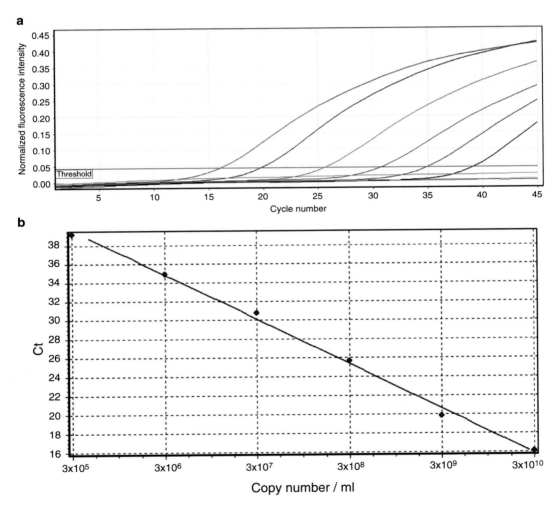

Fig. 1 Real-time RT-PCR assay for ECoV detection used as a quantitative RT-PCR (qRT-PCR): partial M gene amplification of tenfold serial dilution of RNA transcript from ECoV-NC99 strain. (a) Amplification plot of normalized fluorescence intensity versus number of PCR cycles. The X-axis represents the cycle number of the quantitative "M qRT-PCR" assay and the Y-axis, the normalized fluorescence intensity. (b) Standard curve for quantitative analysis of ECoV. The threshold cycle (Ct) is the number of PCR cycles requires for the fluorescent intensity of the reaction to predefine the threshold. The Ct is inversely proportional to the concentration of the input target (from 3×10^{10} to 3×10^5 copy per ml). A linear quantitative detection range with a correlation coefficient (R^2) of 0.997 was obtained with an efficiency of 63 %

4   Notes

1. 1× PBS buffer can be stored at room temperature for 6 months.

2. Two other kits have also been used for RNA extraction from clinical fecal and respiratory samples: the High Pure RNA isolation Kit (Roche®) with 200 μl of clinical sample and a 50 μl final elution volume; and the Mag Attract Viral RNA M48 Kit (Qiagen®), using the BioRobot M48 automated machine (Qiagen®) with 300 μl of clinical sample and a 65 μl final elution volume.

3. Primers and probe used in these assays are perfectly matched with the sequences deduced from the original ECoV-NC99 strain (EF446615) [13].

4. The RT-PCR has also been validated on the SmartCycler II® real-time PCR system (Cepheid®) with the same RT-PCR thermal cycling conditions.

5. The "M qRT-PCR" should be tested with an internal quality control for viral diagnosis in order to exclude false negatives due to possible inhibition.

6. A RNA transcript (10^5 copy/μl) deduced from M gene sequence of ECoV-NC99 strain has been used as positive control.

Acknowledgments

We acknowledge French equine practitioners and the LABEO Frank Duncombe Laboratory for providing fecal and respiratory samples needful to develop this real-time RT-PCR.

References

1. Woo PC, Lau SK, Huang Y, Yuen KY (2009) Coronavirus diversity, phylogeny and interspecies jumping. Exp Biol Med (Maywood) 234(10):1117–1127

2. Guy JS, Breslin JJ, Breuhaus B, Vivrette S, Smith LG (2000) Characterization of a coronavirus isolated from a diarrheic foal. J Clin Microbiol 38(12):4523–4526

3. Oue Y, Ishihara R, Edamatsu H, Morita Y, Yoshida M, Yoshima M et al (2011) Isolation of an equine coronavirus from adult horses with pyrogenic and enteric disease and its antigenic and genomic characterization in comparison with the NC99 strain. Vet Microbiol 150(1–2):41–48

4. Oue Y, Morita Y, Kondo T, Nemoto M (2013) Epidemic of equine coronavirus at Obihiro Racecourse, Hokkaido, Japan in 2012. J Vet Med Sci 75(9):1261–1265

5. Pusterla N, Mapes S, Wademan C, White A, Ball R, Sapp K et al (2013) Emerging outbreaks associated with equine coronavirus in adult horses. Vet Microbiol 162(1):228–231

6. Miszczak F, Tesson V, Kin N, Dina J, Balasuriya UB, Pronost S et al (2014) First detection of equine coronavirus (ECoV) in Europe. Vet Microbiol 171(1-2):206–209

7. Pusterla N, Holzenkaempfer N, Mapes S, Kass P (2015) Prevalence of equine coronavirus in

nasal secretions from horses with fever and upper respiratory tract infection. Vet Rec 177:289

8. Fielding CL, Higgins JK, Higgins JC, McIntosh S, Scott E, Giannitti F et al (2015) Disease associated with equine coronavirus infection and high case fatality rate. J Vet Intern Med 29(1):307–310

9. Magdesian KG, Dwyer RM, Arguedas MG (2014) Viral diarrhea. In: Sellon DC, Long MT (eds) Equine infectious diseases, 2nd edn. Elsevier, St. Louis, pp 198–203

10. Nemoto M, Morita Y, Niwa H, Bannai H, Tsujimura K, Yamanaka T et al (2015) Rapid detection of equine coronavirus by reverse transcription loop-mediated isothermal amplification. J Virol Methods 215–216:13–6

11. Davis E, Rush BR, Cox J, DeBey B, Kapil S (2000) Neonatal enterocolitis associated with coronavirus infection in a foal: a case report. J Vet Diagn Invest 12(2):153–156

12. Slovis NM, Elam J, Estrada M, Leutenegger CM (2013) Infectious agents associated with diarrhoea in neonatal foals in central Kentucky: a comprehensive molecular study. Equine Vet J 46(3):311–316

13. Zhang J, Guy JS, Snijder EJ, Denniston DA, Timoney PJ, Balasuriya UB (2007) Genomic characterization of equine coronavirus. Virology 369(1):92–104

Chapter 9

Detection of Bovine Coronavirus by Conventional Reverse Transcription Polymerase Chain Reaction

Amauri Alcindo Alfieri, Alice Fernandes Alfieri, and Elisabete Takiuchi

Abstract

Bovine coronavirus (BCoV) is an economically significant cause of enteric and respiratory diseases in cattle throughout the world. BCoV is a known cause of neonatal calf diarrhea, winter dysentery in adult cattle, and respiratory disorders in cattle of all ages. In this chapter, we describe a simple and efficient protocol for total nucleic acids extraction to be used in conventional RT-PCR assay. This is a technique used routinely in our virology laboratory to detect BCoV from stool and nasopharyngeal samples of cattle.

Key words Bovine coronavirus, RT-PCR, Clinical diagnosis, Stool samples, Nasopharyngeal samples

1 Introduction

Bovine coronavirus (BCoV) is a member of the order *Nidovirales*, *Coronaviridae* family, which was recently classified as member of the specie *Betacoronavirus 1* in the genus *Betacoronavirus* [1].

BCoV are frequently circulating in cattle farms worldwide, causing both enteric and respiratory disease in calves and adult cattle [2]. Because the respiratory and enteric disorders are similar to the other infectious diseases, a specific test is needed for a conclusive diagnosis of BCoV infection. Besides sensitive tests are required to detect BCoV especially at early or late stages of disease when they have low levels of viral shedding.

The current methods used for the diagnosis of BCoV consist mostly of the detection of viral RNA by conventional (RT-PCR) and real-time reverse transcription polymerase chain reaction (qRT-PCR) [3–6]. Recently, isothermal nucleic acid amplification techniques, such as recombinase polymerase amplification (RPA) assay and reverse transcription loop-mediated isothermal amplification (RT-LAMP), have been developed for rapid detection of BCoV [7, 8]. However, there are still few reports evaluating

Leyi Wang (ed.), *Animal Coronaviruses*, Springer Protocols Handbooks,
DOI 10.1007/978-1-4939-3414-0_9, © Springer Science+Business Media New York 2016

these new assays in large-scale epidemiological studies of BCoV infections.

In this chapter, we describe a sensitive and specific conventional RT-PCR assay that has been successfully applied for diagnosis of both enteric and respiratory bovine coronaviruses [9–12].

2   Materials

2.1   RNA Extraction

1. Sodium dodecyl sulfate (SDS) 10 %.
2. Ultrapure phenol–chloroform–isoamyl alcohol (25:24:1, v/v) (Invitrogen).
3. Silicon Dioxide (SiO_2) (Sigma).
4. Guanidine isothiocyanate (GuSCn) (Invitrogen).
5. Acetone PA.
6. Ethanol solution 70 % (in water).
7. Diethylpyrocarbonate (DEPC)-treated water (Invitrogen).
8. EDTA.
9. Hydrochloric acid 32 %—HCl 32 % (Sigma).
10. Triton X-100 (Invitrogen).
11. Tris (hydroxymethyl)aminomethane (TRIS).
12. Lysis buffer L6.
13. Washing buffer L2.

2.2   Clinical Samples (See Note 1)

Fecal samples: The samples were prepared either as 10 % (w/v) suspensions of solid or semisolid feces in 0.01 M phosphate-buffered saline (PBS) pH 7.2 (137 mM NaCl; 3 mM KCl; 8 mM Na_2HPO_4; 15 mM KH_2PO_4) or as 50 % (v/v) suspensions of liquid feces in 0.01 M PBS and centrifuged at $3000 \times g$ for 15 min at 4 °C. The supernatant is transferred to a sterile tube. Separate an aliquot of 400 µl for RNA extraction.

Nasopharyngeal swab samples: the tip of swab containing nasopharyngeal secretions is soaked in 1 ml of sterile saline solution or 0.01 M PBS. The swab is vortex-mixed for 15 s and then discarded. Centrifuge at $3000 \times g$ for 15 min at 4 °C. The supernatant is transferred to a sterile tube. Separate an aliquot of 450 µl for RNA extraction.

2.3   Preparing Reagent and Solutions Used for RNA Extraction

2.3.1   Silica Hydration Process

Silica suspension is prepared as described by Boom et al. [13] with minor modifications.

1. Suspend six grams of silicon dioxide (SiO_2) in 50 ml of sterile distilled water in a glass graduated cylinder.
2. Slowly stir and keep at rest at room temperature for 24 h for the silica coarse particles to settle.

3. Remove and discard 43 ml of the supernatant from the top with vacuum suction or pipette. Then, resuspend the silica by adding 50 ml of sterile distilled water.

4. Slowly stir and leave for 5 h.

5. Remove and discard 44 ml of the supernatant from the top with vacuum suction or pipette.

6. Add 60 µl of concentrated HCl (32 % w/v) to adjust pH (pH = 2.0).

7. Mix the final content (resulting suspension of silica coarse) and divide into small aliquots (4 ml) into glass bottles with autoclavable cap, tightly closed.

8. Sterilize in an autoclave at 121 °C for 20 min. Store at 4 °C.

2.4 Prepare of Lysis Buffer L6 and Washing Buffer L2

Prepare the following fresh solutions before preparing lysis buffer:

2.4.1 0.1 M Tris–HCl (pH 6.4)

Dissolve 2.67 g of TRIS in 180 ml of distilled water. Add HCl 32 % to adjust the pH to 6.4. Stir vigorously on a magnetic stirrer. Fill up to volume 220 ml with distilled water and set aside at room temperature until use.

2.4.2 0.2 M EDTA (pH 8.0)

Add 1.86 g of EDTA in 15 ml of distilled water. Adjust the pH to 8.0 with NaOH. Fill up to volume 25 ml with distilled water and set aside at room temperature until use (*see* **Note 2**).

2.4.3 Lysis Buffer L6

1. Dissolve 120 g of GuSCN in 100 ml of 0.1 M Tris–HCl (pH 6.4) in a beaker.

2. Add 22 ml of a 0.2 M EDTA solution (pH 8.0).

3. Add 2.6 g of Triton X-100.

4. Homogenize vigorously the solution (*see* **Note 3**).

5. Transfer the solution into a glass bottle with autoclavable cap.

6. Sterilize in an autoclave at 121 °C for 20 min. Store at 4 °C (*see* **Note 4**).

2.4.4 Washing Buffer L2

1. Dissolve 120 g of GuSCN in 100 ml of 0.1 M Tris–HCl (pH 6.4) in a beaker.

2. Homogenize vigorously the solution (*see* **Note 3**).

3. Transfer the solution into a glass bottle with autoclavable cap.

4. Sterilize in an autoclave at 121 °C for 20 min. Store at 4 °C.

2.5 Reverse Transcription

1. Moloney Murine Leukemia Virus Reverse Transcriptase (M-MLV RT), 200 U/µl (Invitrogen).

2. 5× First-Strand Buffer: 250 mM Tris–HCl (pH 8.3), 375 mM KCl, 15 mM $MgCl_2$ (Invitrogen).

3. 0.1 M dithiothreitol (DTT) (Invitrogen).

4. 20 μM reverse primer BCoV2: 5′-TGTGGGTGCGAGTT CTGC-3′ (nt 940–957).

5. Deoxynucleotide triphosphates (dNTP) mix, 10 mM each (Invitrogen).

6. DEPC-treated water (Invitrogen).

7. Thermocycler (Applied Biosystems).

2.6 Polymerase Chain Reaction

1. Platinum *Taq*DNA polymerase, 5 U/μl (Invitrogen).

2. 10× PCR buffer (Invitrogen).

3. 50 mM MgCl$_2$ solution (Invitrogen).

4. Deoxynucleotide triphosphates (dNTP) mix, 10 mM each.

5. 20 μM PCR forward primer, BCoV1: 5′-CGATGAGGCTA TTCCGAC-3′ (nt 504–521).

6. 20 μM PCR reverse primer, BCoV2: 5′-TGTGGGTGCG AGTTCTGC-3′ (nt 940-957).

7. Thermocycler (Applied Biosystems).

2.7 Semi-nested Polymerase Chain Reaction

1. Platinum *Taq*DNA polymerase, 5 U/μl (Invitrogen).

2. 10× PCR buffer (Invitrogen).

3. 50 mM MgCl$_2$ solution (Invitrogen).

4. Deoxynucleotide triphosphates (dNTP) mix, 10 mM each.

5. 20 μM PCR forward primer, BCoV3: 5′-TTGCTAGTCTTGT TCTGGC-3′ (nt 707–725).

6. 20 μM PCR reverse primer, BCoV2: 5′-TGTGGGTGCGAG TTCTGC-3′ (nt 940-957).

7. Thermocycler (Applied Biosystems).

2.8 Gel electrophoresis

1. 1× TRIS–borate–EDTA buffer pH 8.0 (0.89 M TRIS; 0.89 M boric acid; 0.02 M EDTA).

2. UltraPure agarose (Invitrogen).

3. 123 bp DNA ladder markers (Invitrogen).

4. Ethidium bromide, 10 mg/ml.

5. Agarose gel electrophoresis system (Apelex).

6. Power supply (Apelex).

7. Gel Documentation and Analysis System (Kodak).

8. Gel loading buffer (6×): 10 mM Tris–HCl (pH 7.6), 0.03 % bromophenol blue, 0.03 % xylene cyanol, 60 % glycerol, and 60 mM EDTA.

3   Methods

The protocols described below are routinely used for clinical diagnosis of BCoV in cases of neonatal diarrhea, winter dysentery in adult cattle, and respiratory syndrome in cattle of all ages [9, 10].

Firstly, we describe how to obtain high quality nucleic acid total for routine molecular biology applications such as PCR and sequencing. We present an efficient and reproducible protocol for extracting RNA from feces and nasopharyngeal swab samples for BCoV diagnosis. This protocol, which we call phenol chloroform silica method, is based on cellular lysis and protein denaturation by SDS and phenol–chloroform–isoamyl alcohol treatment followed by nucleic acid purification by the guanidinium thiocyanate and silica [14]. Guanidinium thiocyanate is an excellent protein denaturant and hence very effective in inactivating nucleases. Using this protocol extraction it is possible to obtain high quality of RNA in the laboratory on a routine basis without the need for expensive commercial kits extractions.

For RT-PCR assay we chose the N gene because it is highly conserved among BCoV strains (*see* **Note 5**). Also it is known that the N protein is the most abundant antigen in coronavirus-infected cells because its RNA template is the smallest and it has the most abundant sgRNA (subgenomic RNA) during transcription [15]. This indicates that there is more available RNA for the N gene than for the other BCoV protein genes. Consequently, detection of the N gene RNA might be advantageous due to its high abundance in cells, facilitating a high sensitivity of the diagnostic technique.

3.1   RNA Extraction

1. Transfer 450 µl of the fecal or nasopharyngeal suspensions into a 1.5 ml polypropylene microtube. Include at least one positive control (HRT-18 cell culture-adapted BCoV Mebus strain or BCoV wild type strains) and one negative control (DEPC-treated water) in all the RNA extraction procedures.

2. Add 50 µl of SDS 10 % to a final concentration of 1 % (v/v).

3. Vortex for 5 s and incubate in a water bath at 56 °C for 30 min.

4. Add an equal volume (500 µl) of ultrapure phenol–chloroform–isoamyl alcohol to the microtube (*see* **Note 6**). For nasopharyngeal swab samples the treatment with phenol–chloroform–isoamyl alcohol (**steps 2–5**) are not performed.

5. Vortex vigorously for 20 s to mix the phases and incubate in a water bath at 56 °C for 15 min.

6. Centrifuge at $10,000 \times g$ for 10 min to separate the phases (upper aqueous phase, interface, and lower organic phase).

7. Use a micropipette to remove the aqueous phase (upper aqueous phase) into a new 1.5 ml polypropylene microtube. Discard the

microtube containing the interface (between the organic and aqueous phases) and organic phase (lower) (*see* **Notes** 7 and **8**).

8. Add 30 μl of hydrated silica (*see* **Note 9**).

9. Add 900 μl of lysis buffer L6.

10. Vortex vigorously for 20 s.

11. Place the microtubes in a rack and then incubate on an orbital shaker for 30 min at room temperature.

12. Briefly centrifuge the microtubes at $10,000 \times g$ for 30 s to pellet the silica resin.

13. Gently discard the supernatant by inversion (*see* **Note 10**).

14. Add 500 μl of ice-cold washing buffer L2 to the pellet. Vortex for 5 s to resuspend the silica pellet.

15. Briefly centrifuge the microtubes at $10,000 \times g$ for 30 s to pellet the silica resin.

16. Gently discard the supernatant by inversion (*see* **Note 10**).

17. Once again, add 500 μl of ice cold washing buffer L2 to the pellet. Vortex for 5 s to resuspend the silica resin. Repeat **steps** 13 and 14.

18. Add 1 ml of ice-cold ethanol 70 % to the silica pellet. Vortex for 5 s to resuspend the silica pellet.

19. Briefly centrifuge the microtubes at $10,000 \times g$ for 30 s to pellet the silica resin.

20. Gently discard the supernatant by inversion (*see* **Note 10**).

21. Once again add 1 ml of ice cold ethanol 70 % to the pellet. Vortex for 5 s to resuspend the silica resin. Repeat **steps** 17 and 18.

22. Add 1 ml of ice-cold acetone PA to the silica pellet. Vortex for 5 s to resuspend the silica pellet.

23. Centrifuge the microtubes at $10,000 \times g$ for 60 s to pellet the silica resin.

24. Gently discard the supernatant by inversion (*see* **Note 10**).

25. Place the microtubes with open lids in an inverted position over a clean filter paper to drain off the acetone excess.

26. Return the tubes to their normal position and keep them with lids open in a thermoblock (dry block heater) at 56 °C for 15 min to evaporate the acetone and dry the silica pellet.

27. Add 50 μl of DEPC water. Vortex for 5 s to resuspend the silica pellet.

28. Incubate the microtubes with the lids closed in a water bath at 56 °C for 15 min to elute nucleic acid from the silica resin.

29. Centrifuge the microtubes at $10,000 \times g$ for 2 min to pellet the silica resin.

30. Remove the supernatant (nucleic acid eluted) with a micropipette into a new 0.5 ml polypropylene microtube. Discard the microtube containing the silica pellet.

31. Store the eluted nucleic acid at –20 or –80 °C until use (*see* **Note 11**).

3.2 Reverse Transcription (See Note 12)

1. Prepare a reverse transcription (RT) master mix in a volume sufficient for the number of reactions plus 1 in a sterile 1.5 ml polypropylene microtube (label it "RT mix"). The volume of each RT reagent per reaction and the initial and final concentrations are shown in Table 1.

2. Vortex and centrifuge the tube briefly. Keep the microtube "RT mix" on an ice bath until use.

3. Label appropriately the 0.5 μl polypropylene microtubes with the sample identification.

4. Add to each microtube 5 μl of the corresponding sample (eluted RNA), 1 μl of reverse primer BCoV2 and 4 μl of DEPC-treated water.

5. Incubate the microtubes at 97 °C in a heat block for 4 min.

6. Immediately after denaturing place on ice for at least 5 min.

7. Add 10 μl of "RT mix" solution into each microtube.

8. Vortex and centrifuge the tubes briefly.

9. In a thermocycler, incubate the microtubes at 42 °C for 30 min, inactivate the transcription reaction at 95 °C for 5 min and then chill the samples on ice bath.

10. Store the cDNA samples at –20 °C until use.

Table 1
Components of reverse transcription reaction

Reagent	Volume per reaction (μl)	Volume mix for N reactions (μl)	Final concentration
5× First strand buffer	4	$4 \times N$	1×
0.1 mM DTT	2	$2 \times N$	0.01 mM
10 mM dNTP	1	N	0.5 mM
MMLV reverse transcriptase (200 U/μl)	0.5	$0.5 \times N$	100 U/reaction
Water	2.5	$2.5 \times N$	–
Total volume of RT master mix	10	$10 \times N$	–

3.3 PCR Assay

1. Prepare a PCR master mix in a volume sufficient for the number of reactions plus 1 in a sterile 1.5 ml polypropylene microtube and label it "PCR mix." The volume of each PCR reagent per reaction and the initial and final concentrations are shown in Table 2.

2. Vortex and centrifuge the tube briefly. Keep the "PCR mix" on ice bath.

3. Dispense 42 μl of the "PCR mix" into separate 0.5 polypropylene microtube and label the tubes accordingly.

4. Add 8 μl of cDNA generated from the reverse transcription reactions into the correspondent tubes.

5. Vortex and centrifuge the tubes briefly.

6. Run the PCR under the conditions shown in Table 3.

Table 2
Components of the PCR assay

Reagent	Volume per reaction (μl)	Volume mix for N reactions (μl)	Final concentration
10× First strand buffer	7.5	$7.5 \times N$	1.5×
$MgCl_2$, 50 mM	2	$2 \times N$	2 mM
dNTP, 10 mM	4	$4 \times N$	0.8 mM
Reverse primer BCoV2 (20 μM)	1	N	0.4 μM
Forward primer BCoV1 (20 μM)	1	N	0.4 μM
DNA polymerase (5 U/μl)	0.5	$0.5 \times N$	2.5 U/reaction
Water	26	$26 \times N$	–
Total	42	$42 \times N$	–

N = number of 0.2 ml tubes

Table 3
Conditions for PCR assay

Step	Temperature (°C)	Time
1. Heat activation	94	4 min
2. Thermal cycling (40 cycles)		
Denaturing step	94	1 min
Annealing step	55	1 min
Extension	72	1 min
3. Final extension	72	7 min
4. Soak	4	∞

*3.4 Semi-nested
PCR Assay*

1. Prepare a SN-PCR master mix in a volume sufficient for the number of reactions plus 1 in a sterile 1.5 ml polypropylene microtube and label it "SN-PCR mix". The volume of each PCR reagent per reaction and the initial and final concentration are shown in Table 4. Vortex and centrifuge the tube briefly. Keep the "SN-PCR mix" on ice bath.

2. Dispense 47 μl of the "SN-PCR mix" into separate 0.5 polypropylene microtube and label the tubes accordingly.

3. Add 3 μl of the first amplification product (PCR assay) into the correspondent tubes.

4. Vortex and centrifuge the tubes briefly.

5. Run the SN-PCR under the conditions shown in Table 5.

Table 4
Components of the semi-nested PCR assay

Reagent	Volume per reaction (μl)	Volume mix for N reactions (μl)	Final concentration
10× First strand buffer	5	$5 \times N$	1×
MgCl$_2$, 50 mM	2	$2 \times N$	2 mM
dNTP, 10 mM	4	$4 \times N$	0.8 mM
Reverse primer BCoV2 (20 μM)	1	N	0.4 μM
Forward primer BCoV3 (20 μM)	1	N	0.4 μM
DNA polymerase (5 U/μl)	0.5	$0.5 \times N$	2.5 U/reaction
Water	33.5	$33.5 \times N$	–
Total	47	$47 \times N$	–

N = number of 0.2 ml tubes

Table 5
Conditions for the semi-nested PCR assay

Step	Temperature (°C)	Time
1. Heat activation	94	4 min
2. Thermal cycling (30 cycles)		
Denaturing step	94	1 min
Annealing step	55	1 min
Extension	72	1 min
3. Final extension	72	7 min
4. Soak	4	∞

6. After the run, analyze the SN-PCR products by gel electrophoresis. Alternatively, the products can be kept at −20 °C for short-term storage.

3.5 Agarose Gel Electrophoresis

1. Prepare 2 % agarose gel by weighing out 2 g de agarose powder (for gel-tray dimension 14 × 10 × 0.7 cm).Add it into a 250 ml Erlenmeyer flask containing 100 ml 1× TBE buffer.

2. Heat the agarose powder and electrophoresis buffer in a microwave oven until the agarose is completely melted.

3. Let agarose solution cool down to approximately 55 °C.

4. Add 5 μl of ethidium bromide (10 mg/ml) to a final concentration of approximately 0.5 μg/ml (*see* **Notes 13–15**).

5. Pour the solution into a sealed gel casting tray containing a gel comb.

6. Let sit for at least 30 min to solidify at room temperature (the solidified gel is opaque in appearance).

7. Remove the seal and comb. Place the gel and the plastic tray horizontally into the electrophoresis chamber with the wells at the cathode side.

8. Cover the gel with 1× TBE buffer.

9. Pipet 0.5 μl of the DNA markers, 2 μl of 6× gel loading dye and 8 μl de water on a Parafilm sheet and mix well (pipetting up and down).

10. Pipet 10 μl of the SN-PCR products and 2 μl of 6× gel loading dye on a Parafilm sheet and mix well (pipetting up and down).

11. Pipet the samples into the wells.

12. Close the lid and connect the power leads on the electrophoresis apparatus.

13. Turn on power supply and apply a voltage of 80–100 V. Run the gel for approximately 40 min.

14. Turn off the power supply when the tracking dye has migrated a sufficient distance.

15. Remove the cover and retrieve the gel (*see* **Note 16**).

16. Place the gel on an ultraviolet transilluminator. Switch on the power of the gel photo-documentation machine (*see* **Note 17**).

17. Adjust the position of the gel and record the results. The size of the expected product for BCoV is 454 bp and 251 bp for the first and second round of amplification, respectively.

4 Notes

1. Clinical samples must be store at 4 °C for up to 48 h or frozen or −80 °C for longer periods of time. The sensitivity of the PCR could be reduced if you repeat freezing and thawing of fecal samples. Store samples in multiple small aliquots to avoid repeated freeze–thaw cycles which accelerate degradation of nucleic acids, especially RNA.

2. The disodium salt of EDTA will not dissolve until the pH of the solution is adjusted to 8.0 by the addition of NaOH.

3. Dissolution of GuSCN is facilitated by heating in a 60–65 °C water bath under continuous shaking.

4. Buffers L6 and L2 are stable for at least 3 weeks at room temperature in the dark [13].

5. The three primers used in SN-PCR were designed from the highly conserved region of the N gene of the Mebus strain (GenBank accession number U00735).

6. Phenol is highly corrosive and can cause severe burns to skin. Personal protective equipment such as gloves, safety glasses, and a lab coat are essentials whenever working with phenol.

7. Be careful not to transfer any of the protein at the interphase.

8. Phenol and chloroform are considered hazardous chemicals by waste environment protection agencies and similar bodies around the world. Discard phenol–chloroform–isoamyl alcohol waste in a properly labeled container. For more information regarding hazardous waste management, contact your state hazardous waste agency.

9. Be careful to stir the tube containing hydrated silica before use to resuspend settled silica.

10. Be careful not to disturb the silica pellet when discarding the supernatant. Attention: GuSCN-containing waste should be collected in a strong alkaline solution (10 N NaOH).

11. If you perform the RT-PCR on the same day, RNA extraction can be conserved at 4 °C. For a longer conservation period, RNA must be stored at −80 °C.

12. It is recommended to carry out the cDNA synthesis immediately after the RNA preparation. Being more stable than RNA, the storage of a first-strand cDNA is less critical.

13. Alternatively, the gel can be stained after DNA separation by electrophoresis. Place the gel into a container filled with 100 ml of TBE running buffer and 5 µl of ethidium bromide. Let the gel soak in this solution for 20–30 min. Wash the gel briefly with water before visualization under UV light.

14. Ethidium bromide is mutagenic and moderately toxic and must be handled with care. Wear a lab coat, eye protection, and gloves when working with this chemical.

15. Liquid (running buffer) and solid (agarose gel, gloves, tips) waste contaminated with ethidium bromide must be managed as a hazardous waste. No liquids should be placed in the containers with the solid wastes. For more information regarding hazardous waste management, contact your state hazardous waste agency.

16. DNA will diffuse within the gel over time. Therefore, examination or photography should take place shortly after cessation of electrophoresis.

17. Exposure to UV light can cause severe skin and eye damage. Wear safety glasses and close the photography hood before turning on the UV transilluminator. Be certain to turn off UV light immediately after gel image is captured.

Acknowledgments

Alfieri, A.A. and Alfieri A.F. are recipients of the CNPq fellowships.

References

1. de Groot RJ, Baker SC, Baric R et al (2011) Family Coronaviridae. In: King AMQ, Adams MJ, Carstens EB et al (eds) Virus taxonomy, classification and nomenclature of viruses. Ninth report of the international committee on taxonomy of viruses. Elsevier Academic Press, Philadelphia, pp 806–828

2. Boileau MJ, Kapil S (2010) Bovine coronavirus associated syndromes. Vet Clin North Am Food Anim Pract 26:123–146. doi:10.1016/j.cvfa.2009.10.003

3. Takiuchi E, Stipp D, Alfieri AF et al (2006) Improved detection of bovine coronavirus N gene in faeces of calves infected naturally by a semi-nested PCR assay and an internal control. J Virol Methods 131:148–154. doi:10.1016/j.jviromet.2005.08.005

4. Decaro N, Elia G, Campolo M et al (2008) Detection of bovine coronavirus using a TaqMan-based real-time RT-PCR assay. J Virol Methods 151:167–171. doi:10.1016/j.jviromet.2008.05.016

5. Decaro N, Campolo M, Desario C et al (2008) Respiratory disease associated with bovine coronavirus infection in cattle herds in Southern Italy. J Vet Diagn Invest 20:28–32. doi:10.1177/104063870802000105

6. Amer HM, Almajhdi FN (2011) Development of a SYBR Green I based real-time RT-PCR assay for detection and quantification of bovine coronavirus. Mol Cell Probes 25:101–107. doi:10.1016/j.mcp.2011.03.001

7. Qiao J, Meng Q, Cai X et al (2011) Rapid detection of Betacoronavirus 1 from clinical fecal specimens by a novel reverse transcription loop-mediated isothermal amplification assay. J Vet Diagn Invest 24:174–177. doi:10.1177/1040638711425937

8. Amer HM, Abd El Wahed A, Ma S et al (2013) A new approach for diagnosis of bovine coronavirus using a reverse transcription recombinase polymerase amplification assay. J Virol Methods 193:337–340. doi:10.1016/j.jviromet.2013.06.027

9. Stipp DT, Barry AF, Alfieri AF et al (2009) Frequency of BCoV detection by a semi-nested PCR assay in faeces of calves from Brazilian cattle herds. Trop Anim Health Prod 41:1563–1567. doi:10.1007/s11250-009-9347-2

10. Takiuchi E, Aline AF, Alfieri AF et al (2009) An outbreak of winter dysentery caused by bovine coronavirus in a high-production dairy cattle herd from a tropical country. Trop

Anim Health Prod 52:57–61. doi:10.1590/s1516-89132009000700008

11. Fulton RW, Blood KS, Panciera RJ et al (2009) Lung pathology and infectious agents in fatal feedlot pneumonias and relationship with mortality, disease onset, and treatments. J Vet Diag Invest 21:464–477. doi:10.1177/104063870902100407

12. Fulton RW, Step DL, Wahrmund J et al (2011) Bovine coronavirus (BCV) infections in transported commingled beef cattle and sole-source ranch calves. Can J Vet Res 75:191–199

13. Boom R, Sol CJ, Salimans MM et al (1990) Rapid and simple method for purification of nucleic acids. J Clin Microbiol 28:495–503

14. Alfieri AA, Parazzi ME, Takiuchi E et al (2006) Frequency of group A rotavirus in diarrhoeic calves in Brazilian cattle herds, 1998–2002. Trop Anim Health Prod 38:521–526. doi:10.1007/s11250-006-4349-9

15. Hofmann MA, Sethna PB, Brian DA (1990) Bovine coronavirus mRNA replication continues throughout persistent infection in cell culture. J Virol 64:4108–4114

Chapter 10

Real-Time Reverse Transcription Polymerase Chain Reaction for Rapid Detection of Transmissible Gastroenteritis Virus

Ramesh Vemulapalli

Abstract

Transmissible gastroenteritis (TGE) is a highly contagious disease of pigs caused by the TGE virus (TGEV). Rapid detection of the virus in the affected pigs' feces is critical for controlling the disease outbreaks. The real-time RT-PCR assay described in this chapter can quickly detect the presence of TGEV in fecal samples with high sensitivity and specificity.

Key words TGE virus, Real-time RT-PCR, Feces, Pigs

1 Introduction

Transmissible gastroenteritis (TGE) is a highly contagious, acute viral disease of pigs [1]. TGE can affect pigs of all ages, but the disease severity and mortality rate are high in piglets under 2 weeks of age. The causative agent is TGE virus (TGEV), a coronavirus that primarily infects and replicates in the epithelial cells of pig intestines. Affected animals shed the virus in their feces. The disease transmission occurs primarily via fecal-oral route [2]. During an outbreak, rapid detection of TGEV in feces is very useful for implementing the disease management practices in a timely manner. Any TGEV-specific diagnostic assay must be able to differentiate it from porcine respiratory coronavirus (PRCV), a natural mutant of TGEV with truncated spike protein and altered cell tropism towards respiratory epithelial cells [3]. PRCV mostly causes mild or subclinical respiratory disease. However, in some PRCV-infected pigs, the virus can be shed in the feces [4]. Real-time PCR-based assays are well suited for rapid, specific, and sensitive detection of viruses such as TGEV. The real-time RT-PCR assay described here is based on amplification of a conserved region of the spike protein gene of TGEV strains and detection of

Leyi Wang (ed.), *Animal Coronaviruses*, Springer Protocols Handbooks,
DOI 10.1007/978-1-4939-3414-0_10, © Springer Science+Business Media New York 2016

the amplified products using a TaqMan probe [5]. The assay, along with the RNA extraction method described here, can be established in any molecular diagnostic laboratory for detection of TGEV in pig fecal samples [6–8].

2   Materials

2.1   RNA Extraction

1. TRIzol LS Reagent (Invitrogen).
2. RNeasy Mini Kit (Qiagen).
3. Chloroform.
4. Ethanol, 70 and 96–100 %.
5. DNase/RNase-free distilled water.
6. Feces samples from suspected pigs.

2.2   Real-Time RT-PCR

1. OneStep RT-PCR Kit (Qiagen).
2. RNasin Ribonuclease Inhibitor (Promega) or equivalent.
3. 25 mM $MgCl_2$ solution for PCR (Sigma-Aldrich) or equivalent.
4. DNase/RNase-free distilled water.
5. 10 μM Forward primer, 5′-TCTGCTGAAGGTGCTATTAT ATGC-3′.
6. 10 μM Reverse primer, 5′-CCACAATTTGCCTCTGAATTAG AAG-3′.
7. 2.5 μM Probe 5′-(FAM)YAAGGGCTCACCACCTACTACCA CCA(BHQ1)-3′(FAM, 6-carboxyfluorescein; BHQ1, black hole quencher 1; Eurofins MWG Operon).
8. Real-time PCR machine, such as Smart Cycler II (Cepheid), 7300 Real-Time PCR System (Applied Biosystems), or equivalent.
9. PCR reaction tubes suitable for the real-time PCR machine platform.

3   Methods

Preventing contamination of samples and reagents with nucleic acids and nucleases is critical to obtaining accurate and reproducible results with any PCR-based diagnostic assay. It is recommended that the nucleic acid extraction, preparation of master mix, and real-time PCR amplification are performed in three physically separated areas. Each of these areas should have separate set of laboratory instruments and supplies that are to be used only in their assigned location [9]. Including a positive extraction control and a negative extraction control along with each batch of clinical samples is recommended to monitor the efficiency of RNA extraction and potential cross contamination of the samples [9].

3.1 RNA Extraction

PCR inhibitors are often co-extracted with nucleic acids from fecal samples. In our experience, RNA extracted from pig fecal samples using the following method is suitable for TGEV detection using the real-time RT-PCR assay. Other extraction methods that produce PCR inhibitor-free RNA can also be used (*see* **Note 1**). The presence of PCR inhibitors in the extracted can be monitored by using an internal control (*see* **Note 2**).

1. Prepare a 20 % (w/v) suspension of feces in DNase/RNase-free distilled water. Feces in liquid form can be used directly.

2. Transfer 250 μl of the fecal suspension into a 1.5 ml microcentrifuge tube.

3. Add 750 μl of TRIzol LS reagent, briefly vortex the tube for 10 s, and incubate at room temperature for 5 min.

4. Add 200 μl of chloroform to the tube. Vortex the tube for 5 s and incubate at room temperature for 3 min.

5. Centrifuge the tube at $12,000 \times g$ for 10 min.

6. Transfer 600 μl of the top aqueous phase to a new 1.5 ml microcentrifuge tube containing 600 μl of 70 % ethanol and mix by inverting 4–5 times.

7. Transfer 700 μl of the mix to an RNeasy spin column and centrifuge at $8000 \times g$ for 30 s.

8. Transfer the spin column to a new collection tube, and add the remaining mix from **step 6**. Centrifuge at $8000 \times g$ for 30 s.

9. Place the spin column into a new collection tube. Add 700 μl of RW1 buffer to the spin column and centrifuge at $8000 \times g$ for 30 s.

10. Place the spin column into a new collection tube. Add 500 μl of RPE buffer to the spin column and centrifuge at $8000 \times g$ for 30 s (*see* **Note 3**).

11. Repeat **step 10** for a second wash of the spin column with RPE buffer.

12. Place the spin column into a new collection tube and centrifuge at $10,000 \times g$ for 1 min to dry the membrane of the column.

13. Place the spin column in a 1.5 ml microcentrifuge tube and add 30 μl of DNase/RNase-free water to the column. Incubate at room temperature for 1 min.

14. Centrifuge at $10,000 \times g$ for 1 min.

15. Discard the spin column and store the eluted RNA at 4 °C if it is used in the real-time RT-PCR assay within 12 h or at −20 °C if it is used after 12 h (*see* **Note 4**).

3.2 Real-Time RT-PCR

1. Turn on the real-time PCR machine. Follow the software directions of the machine manufacturer to confirm that the FAM signal data will be gathered during the amplification. Program the thermal cycle and data collection conditions according to Table 1.

2. Prepare a master mix sufficient for the intended number of samples in a sterile 1.5 ml microcentrifuge tube according to Table 2. Add at least a no-template control (NTC) and a positive amplification control (PAC) to the number required reactions.

3. Close the cap of the microcentrifuge tube. Vortex and centrifuge the tube briefly.

4. Aliquot 20 μl of the master mix into each PCR reaction tube.

Table 1
Thermal cycling conditions

Step		Temperature (°C)	Time
1. Reverse transcription		50	30 min
2. Heat inactivation of reverse transcriptase and activation of Taq DNA polymerase		95	15 min
3. Amplification and detection (45 cycles)	Denaturation	95	15 s
	Annealing and data collection	56	30 s
	Extension	72	15 s

Table 2
Master mix components

Reagent	Volume per reaction (μl)	Final concentration
RNase-free water	6.2	–
5× Qiagen OneStep RT-PCR buffer	5.0	1×
10 mM dNTPs	0.8	0.2 mM
10 μM Forward primer	1.0	0.4 μM
10 μM Reverse primer	3.0	1.2 μM
2.5 μM Probe	1.5	0.15 μM
Ribonuclease inhibitor (13 U/μl)	1.0	13 U/reaction
25 mM MgCl$_2$	0.5	0.5 mM
Qiagen OneStep RT-PCR enzyme mix	1.0	–

5. Add 5 μl of the extracted sample RNA. Add 5 μl of DNase/RNase-free water to the NTC tube. Add 5 μl of RNA extracted from TGEV to the PAC tube.

6. Centrifuge the PCR tubes briefly.

7. Insert the PCR tubes into the real-time PCR machine and start the thermal cycling program.

8. At the completion of the amplification program, examine the amplification curves and the threshold cycles (Ct) of the reactions. The NTC reaction and any other negative control reactions should not generate a Ct value. The PAC reaction and any other expected positive reactions should generate a Ct value as expected based on the template RNA concentration.

4   Notes

1. Magnetic bead-based manual or high-throughput RNA extraction methods (e.g., MagMax Viral RNA Isolation Kit, Life Technologies) are used in our laboratory to extract TGEV and other viral RNA from pig fecal samples.

2. Xeno RNA (Life Technologies) can be used as internal RNA control to monitor the presence of PCR inhibitors and efficiency of RNA extraction.

3. Buffer RPE of the RNeasy Kit is supplied as a concentrate. Follow the manufacturer's direction to prepare the buffer by adding the appropriate volume of 100 % ethanol.

4. For long-term storage, it is recommended that the extracted viral RNA be kept at −80 °C.

References

1. Garwes DJ (1988) Transmissible gastroenteritis. Vet Rec 122:462–463

2. Saif LJ, van Cott JL, Brim TA (1994) Immunity to transmissible gastroenteritis virus and porcine respiratory coronavirus infections in swine. Vet Immunol Immunopathol 43:89–97

3. Rasschaert D, Duarte M, Laude H (1990) Porcine respiratory coronavirus differs from transmissible gastroenteritis virus by a few genomic deletions. J Gen Virol 71:2599–2607

4. Costantini V, Lewis P, Alsop J, Templeton C et al (2004) Respiratory and fecal shedding of porcine respiratory coronavirus (PRCV) in sentinel weaned pigs and sequence of the partial S-gene of the PRCV isolates. Arch Virol 149:957–974

5. Vemulapalli R, Gulani J, Santrich C (2009) A real-time TaqMan® RT-PCR assay with an internal amplification control for rapid detection of transmissible gastroenteritis virus in swine fecal samples. J Virol Methods 162:231–235

6. Huang Y, Harding JCS (2014) Attempted experimental reproduction of porcine periweaning-failure-to-thrive syndrome using tissue homogenates. PLoS One 9:e90065

7. Ojkic D, Hazlett M, Fairles J, Marom A et al (2015) The first case of porcine epidemic diarrhea in Canada. Can Vet J 56:149–152

8. Wang X, Ren W, Nie Y, Cheng L et al (2013) A novel watery diarrhea caused by the co-infection of neonatal piglets with *Clostridium perfringens* type A and *Escherichia coli* (K88, 987P). Vet J 197:812–816

9. Kessler HH, Raggam RB (2012) Quality assurance and quality control in the routine molecular diagnostic laboratory for infectious diseases. Clin Chem Lab Med 50:1153–1159

Chapter 11

An RT-PCR Assay for Detection of Infectious Bronchitis Coronavirus Serotypes

Junfeng Sun and Shengwang Liu

Abstract

Avian infectious bronchitis virus (IBV), a chicken Gammacoronavirus, is a major poultry pathogen, and is probably endemic in all regions with intensive poultry production. Since IBV was first described in 1936, many serotypes and variants of IBV have been isolated worldwide. IBV isolates are capable of infecting a large range of epithelial surfaces of the chicken, involving the respiratory, renal, and reproductive systems; however, the clinical signs are usually not specific for differential diagnoses. Virus isolation is commonly used for diagnosis of IBV infection, which was achieved through passage of clinical materials via the allantoic route of embryos. Currently, more sensitive molecular approaches for the detection of avian pathogens have been developed, including reverse-transcriptase polymerase chain reaction (RT-PCR) and real-time RT-PCR, which are more suitable for use in diagnostic laboratories. In this chapter, we describe a one-step RT-PCR which can be used for detecting most of IBV serotypes in the IBV-infected allantoic fluid and has been used routinely in our laboratories for detection of IBVs.

Key words IBV, RT-PCR, Molecular detection, Diagnosis, Clinical samples

1 Introduction

Infectious bronchitis (IB) is an acute and highly contagious viral disease of chicken caused by the infectious bronchitis virus (IBV). This disease is prevalent throughout the world and affects the performance of both meat-type and egg-laying birds, thereby causing severe economic loss within the poultry industry. IB can affect chickens of all ages and result in respiratory disease, nephritis, proventriculitis, and decrease in egg production and egg quality [1–3]. Furthermore, this disease is often complicated by secondary bacterial infections that cause increased mortality. It may be the most economically important viral respiratory tract disease of chickens in countries and regions where there is no highly pathogenic avian influenza virus or velogenic (highly pathogenic) Newcastle disease virus [4].

Leyi Wang (ed.), *Animal Coronaviruses*, Springer Protocols Handbooks,
DOI 10.1007/978-1-4939-3414-0_11, © Springer Science+Business Media New York 2016

IBV is a *gammacoronavirus* of the subfamily *Coronavirinae*, family *Coronaviridae*, and order *Nidovirales*. The IBV genome is an approximately 27.6-kb linear, non-segmented, positive-sense, single-stranded RNA. The viral genome is 5' capped, with a poly-A tail and the gene organization is 5' UTR-1a/1ab-S-3a-3b-E-M-5a-5b-N-3' UTR. The 5' two-thirds of the IBV genome encodes two polyproteins 1a and 1ab that contain nonstructural proteins which are associated with viral RNA replication and transcription, whereas the 3' one-third encodes four structural proteins: the surface spike glycoprotein (S), and small envelope (E), membrane (M), and nucleocapsid (N) proteins [5].

Virus isolation is the "gold standard" for the diagnosis of IBV infection. Since there is lack of cell lines to support the growth of IBV, 9- to 11-day-old embryo inoculation via the allantoic route is commonly used for virus isolation. The characteristic embryo changes, such as dwarfing, stunting, or curling of embryos, can be observed between 2 and 7 days after the inoculation. This type of diagnosis assay has been used for many years. However, for most of the field samples, several blind passages (more than three times) were needed before typical characteristic embryo changes can be observed, and interpretation of the results was subjective. In addition, this method is time consuming (2–7 days for each passage are needed before embryo lesions can be observed) and expensive (requires a large amount of embryos) [4, 6, 7].

In order to obtain rapid and accurate diagnostic results, more sensitive molecular methods for the detection of IBV have been developed, including reverse-transcriptase polymerase chain reaction (RT-PCR), and real-time RT-PCR [8]. Primer pairs targeting to the 3' untranslated region (UTR), N gene, and the S1 and S2 parts of the S gene of IBV genome have been reported to detect as many as possible, although not all, isolates of IBV [8–12]. Furthermore, the DNA fragment produced from the RT-PCR-based method can be further sequenced for phylogenetic analysis.

The N gene and 3' UTR are the most conserved regions in the genome of IBV serotypes [13]. Furthermore, a nested set of IBV subgenomic mRNAs (sgRNAs) is produced via a discontinuous transcription mechanism, and the N gene and 3' UTR are the most abundant productions during transcription [14, 15]. These characteristics demonstrate that the N gene and 3' UTR of IBV are the appropriate candidates for molecular diagnosis. In our epidemiology surveillance of IBV in China, we have successfully used a set of primers targeting the N gene and 3' UTR to detect IBV in allantoic fluids of embryos inoculated with tissue, oropharyngeal, and cloacal swab samples. In this chapter, we describe the procedures of one-step RT-PCR for the detection of IBV from a range of sample types that were used in our IBV epidemiology surveillance studies. This assay together with virus isolation is designed specifically for the rapid detection of serotypes of IBV from clinical samples.

2 Materials

2.1 Sample Handing

1. 9- to 11-day-old embryonated SPF chicken eggs (*see* **Note 1**).

2. Sterile phosphate-buffered solution (PBS). Store at room temperature.

3. Viral transport medium for swabs (500 ml PBS containing 0.1 g gentamicin, 0.25 g kanamycin, 1.25 mg amphotericin B, and 5 ml equine serum). Store at –20 °C.

4. Oropharyngeal and cloacal swabs and tissue samples from the kidney, proventriculus, trachea, and caecal tonsil from commercial flocks of cockerels, broilers, pullets, layers, and breeders suspected of IBV infection (*see* **Notes 2** and **3**). Store at –70 °C.

5. TissueLyser II (Qiagen, Germany).

2.2 RNA Extraction

1. TRIzol reagents (Invitrogen, Grand Island, New York, USA). Store at 4 °C.

2. RNase-free Water (TaKaRa, Dalian, China). Store at room temperature.

3. Chloroform. Store at room temperature.

4. Isopropyl alcohol. Store at room temperature.

5. 75 % Ethanol (in RNase-free water). Store at –20 °C.

2.3 IBV One-Step RT-PCR

1. The primers are prepared in a stock solution of 100 μM with RNase-free water. A working solution of 10 μM is made for use in the RT-PCR. Store at –20 °C until use.

   Forward primer: N (+) 5′-GACGCCCCAGCGCCAGTCATTA AA-3′.

   Reverse primer: N (–) 5′-ACGCGGAGTACGATCGAGGG TACA-3′ (TaKaRa, Dalian, China) (*see* **Note 4**).

2. TaKaRa PrimeScript One Step RT-PCR Kit Ver.2 containing PrimeScript 1 Step Enzyme Mix, 2 × 1 Step Buffer, and RNase Free dH$_2$O (TaKaRa, Dalian, China). Store all reagents at –20 °C.

3. TaKaRa PCR Thermal Cycler Dice™ Gradient TP600 (TaKaRa, Dalian, China).

2.4 PCR Product Detection and Purification

1. 1× Tris-acetate-EDTA (TAE) buffer. Store at room temperature.

2. Agarose gels (1 % agarose in 1× TAE buffer containing 0.5 μg/ml ethidium bromide).

3. 250 bp DNA Ladder (Dye Plus) (TaKaRa, Dalian, China). Store at 4 °C.

4. ChemiDocMP Imaging System (Bio-Rad, Hercules, CA, USA).

5. E.Z.N.A. Gel Extraction Kit (Omega Bio-Tek, USA). Store at room temperature.

2.5 PCR Product Cloning

1. pMD 18-T Vector Cloning Kit (TaKaRa, Dalian, China). Store at −20 °C.
2. DH5α competent cells kit (TaKaRa, Dalian, China). Store at −70 °C.
3. LB plate containing 100 μg/ml ampicillin, 24 μg/ml X-Gal, and 40 μg/ml IPTG. Store at 4 °C.
4. LB liquid culture medium containing 100 μg/ml ampicillin. Store at 4 °C.
5. Premix Taq (Ex TaqVersion 2.0) (TaKaRa, Dalian, China). Store at −20 °C.

2.6 Sequencing and Sequence Analysis

1. Sequencing: At least three clones were sequenced each time.
2. DNASTAR's Lasergene Sequence Analysis Software.
3. Molecular Evolutionary Genetics Analysis (MEGA) Software.

3 Methods

3.1 Sample Handling

1. Tissue samples: Homogenize the tissue samples as 10 % weight/volume tissue suspensions in PBS by using TissueLyser II (Qiagen, Germany), freeze-thaw three times at −20 °C and room temperature, and then clarify by centrifugation at $1500 \times g$ at 4 °C for 10 min; use 200 μl of the supernatant to inoculate into the allantoic cavity of 9-day-old to 11-day-old SPF embryos. At 3 days after inoculation, take 200 μl allantoic fluid for viral RNA extraction. Store the rest of the sample at −80 °C (*see* **Notes 1, 5–6**).
2. Swab samples: Place the tip of the swab in a 1.5 ml EP tube containing 1 ml viral transport medium. After squeezing the tip of the swap and vortexing, take 200 μl of the solution for embryo inoculation and 200 μl allantoic fluid for subsequent viral RNA extraction at 3 days after inoculation. Store the rest of the sample at −80 °C (*see* **Notes 1, 6**, and **7**).

3.2 RNA Extraction

Viral RNA was extracted from 200 μl of allantoic fluid from embryos that have been inoculated with tissue and oropharyngeal and cloacal swab samples using TRIzol (Invitrogen), which is a reagent that has been used to isolate high quality of total RNA from various types of samples. We followed the manufacturer's instructions with minor changes:

1. Pipette 200 μl allantoic fluid into 1.5 ml RNase-free microcentrifuge tube (*see* **Note 8**).
2. Add 1 ml TRIzol reagent to each tube, and incubate for 5 min at room temperature after vortexing thoroughly.
3. Add 0.2 ml of chloroform per 1 ml of TRIzol reagent. Shake tube vigorously by hand for 15 s.

4. Incubate for 2–3 min at room temperature.

5. Centrifuge the tube at 12,000×g for 15 min at 4 °C.

6. Transfer the aqueous phase into a new RNase-free tube. Avoid disturbing the interphase or organic layer when removing the aqueous phase.

7. Add 0.5 ml of 100 % isopropanol to the aqueous phase, per 1 ml of TRIzol reagent.

8. Incubate at –20 °C for 30 min.

9. Centrifuge the tube at 12,000×g for 15 min at 4 °C.

10. Remove the supernatant, leaving the RNA pellet on the bottom of the tube (*see* **Note 9**).

11. Wash the RNA pellet with 1 ml of 75 % ethanol per 1 ml of TRIzol reagent.

12. Vortex the sample briefly, and then centrifuge the tube at 7500×g for 5 min at 4 °C. Discard the wash.

13. Air-dry the RNA pellet for 5–10 min (*see* **Note 10**).

14. Resuspend the RNA pellet in RNase-free water.

15. (Optional) Incubate the tube in a water bath at 55–60 °C for 10–15 min to increase the solubilization rate.

16. The obtained RNA should be stored at –70 °C or applied directly for subsequent one-step RT-PCR.

3.3 IBV One-Step RT-PCR

1. Detecting a sample for the presence of IBV is performed by amplifying a 1604-bp fragment of the IBV N gene and 3′ UTR using the primer set N (+) and N (–) described in Sect. 2.3. We used a one-step RT-PCR kit throughout the procedure (*see* **Note 11**). Perform all RT-PCR steps on ice. Prepare the following mix for RT-PCR according to the number of samples to be tested: PrimeScript 1 Step Enzyme Mix 2 μl, 2×1 Step Buffer 25 μl, forward primer 1 μl, reverse primer 1 μl, and RNase-free water to 48 μl per reaction (*see* **Note 12**).

2. Add 2 μl RNA sample to the 0.2 ml PCR tube containing 48 μl of RT-PCR mix, leading to a final reaction volume of 50 μl. The reaction is carried out with an initial reverse transcription step at 50 °C for 30 min, followed by PCR activation at 94 °C for 2 min, 30 cycles of amplification (30 s at 94 °C; 30 s at 60 °C; 2 min at 72 °C), and a final extension step at 72 °C for 10 min in PCR Thermal Cycler Dice™ Gradient TP600 (*see* **Notes 13** and **14**).

3.4 PCR Product Detection and Purification

1. Load 4 μl of PCR product mixed with 1 μl loading buffer on a 1 % agarose gel. Load 5 μl 250 bp DNA Ladder on the left side of the gel. Run the gel at 180 V for 20 min. Visualize the bands by illuminating the gel with UV light on the Bio-Rad ChemiDocMP Imaging System (Bio-Rad, Hercules, CA, USA).

2. Determination of the products' fragment size is carried out by comparing the length of the bands to 250 bp DNA Ladder. Samples from which a PCR product of approximately 1600 bp is amplified are presumed to be IBV positive.

3. Extraction and purification of PCR product are performed by using E.Z.N.A. Gel Extraction Kit (Omega Bio-Tek, USA) according to the manufacturer's instructions. The purified PCR products are then used as templates for sequencing. Alternatively, these samples could be stored at −20 °C until use.

3.5 PCR Product Cloning (Optional)

1. Mix 9 μl purified PCR products with 10 μl solution I and 1 μl pMD18-T vector provided by pMD 18-T Vector Cloning Kit (TaKaRa, Dalian, China). Incubate the 20 μl mixture at 16 °C overnight.

2. Thaw a vial of DH5α competent cells on ice.

3. Add 20 μl reaction mixture into the thawed DH5α competent cells; incubate on ice for 30 min after slightly mixing.

4. Heat shock 90 s at 42 °C, and then chill on ice for 2–3 min.

5. Add 1 ml SOC medium provided from the competent cells kit to the transfected cells and incubate at 37 °C with shaking for 1 h.

6. Centrifuge at $1500 \times g$ for 5 min and remove 800 μl supernatant from the tube.

7. Cells were resuspended in the rest of the medium and then spread onto the LB plate containing 100 μg/ml ampicillin, 24 μg/ml X-Gal, and 40 μg/ml IPTG. Incubate the plate at 37 °C overnight in an inverted position.

8. Select and mark white colonies for PCR screening. Use sterile pipette tips to pick the selected colonies and then transfer the tips into tubes with 5 ml LB containing 100 μg/ml ampicillin; incubate these tubes at 37 °C overnight with shaking.

9. Identify the bacteria culture through PCR using forward primer: N (+) and reverse primer: N (−).

   Prepare the following reaction mix for PCR: Premix Taq 12.5 μl, forward primer: N (+) 1 μl, reverse primer: N (−) 1 μl, bacteria culture 1 μl, and sterilized water up to 25 μl. PCR thermocycler is set at the following conditions: 10-min incubation at 94 °C, 30 cycles of 94 °C for 30 s, annealing at 60 °C for 30 s, and 72 °C for 2 min, and a final extension step at 72 °C for 10 min.

10. Agarose gel electrophoresis is used to determine the size of the inserts of these clones according to the procedures described in Sect. 3.4. Clones with the expected product sizes will be selected for sequencing.

3.6 Sequence Analysis

The nucleotide sequences of the IBV serotypes are assembled, aligned, and compared with those of other reference IBV serotypes using DNASTAR's Lasergene Sequence Analysis Software. A Maximum Likelihood tree based on the JTT matrix-based model and 100 bootstrap replicates was built using the MEGA 4.

4 Notes

1. In order to determine the sensitivity of the diagnostic IBV RT-PCR assay, we compared this assay with the current standard test, virus isolation in SPF embryos. A tenfold dilution series of the IBV H120 strain (10^7 EID_{50}) was prepared; 200 μl of each dilution was tested in parallel by both tests. The limit of detection of virus isolation was 0.5×10^1 EID_{50}, while the limit of detection of the RT-PCR was 500 EID_{50}. These results showed that this IBV RT-PCR assay is less sensitive than virus isolation for the IBV-infected allantoic fluid. However, we found that after inoculating tissue and oropharyngeal and cloacal swab samples into the allantoic cavities of 9-day-old to 11-day-old SPF embryos, this IBV RT-PCR assay can efficiently detect the IBV in allantoic fluids, and no extra blind passage is needed. In practice, we have successfully used this assay together with virus isolation, to detect most serotypes of IBV from clinical samples during our epidemiology surveillance of IBV in China.

2. Swab sample collection: IBV isolates can infect a large range of epithelial surfaces including respiratory tissues and non-respiratory tissues of chicken. Since the primary target tissue for IBV is the respiratory tract, oropharyngeal swabs is a good choice for detection of IBV especially in the early stages of infection due to that IBV persists in the respiratory tract for a relatively short time after infection. For collecting oropharyngeal swab samples, insert swab into the bird's throat and leave it in place for a few seconds to absorb secretions.

   It is considered that replication of IBV in intestinal tract normally does not cause clinical disease, although it does result in faecal excretion of the virus. The excretion of IBV in the faeces may be associated with apparent long-term persistence of IBV in chicken flocks. Therefore, cloacal swab is the material of choice to detect IBV. For collecting cloacal swab samples, insert swab into the bird's cloaca and stir for a few seconds to stick faeces.

3. The selection of tissue material for IBV isolation or detection is critical because IBV can affect many tissues, involving the respiratory, renal, and reproductive systems. In our previous study, we have successfully detected the IBV from kidney,

proventriculus, trachea, and caecal tonsil from commercial chickens. In practice, trachea tissue can be chosen for IBV detection when chicken showed respiratory symptoms. In addition, kidney and caecal tonsil are candidate materials when investigating kidney infection or declined egg laying performance. If swelling of the proventriculus, the characteristic changes of infected chickens, occurs, proventriculus can be selected as sample for IBV detection.

4. In order to detect as many IBV serotypes as possible, N protein genes from 228 IBV strains available in GenBank were aligned using the MegAlign application in the Lasergene software package [16]. The forward primer N (+) targeting a conserved region of IBV N gene and reverse primer N (−) targeting the conversed 3′ UTR of the IBV genome were designed. We have successfully detected the Massachusetts, 4/91, LX4, CK/CH/LSC/99I, CK/CH/LDL/97I, and Connecticut type of IBV serotypes by using this pair of primers.

   The Georgia 98, Arkansas, and Florida (isolated from USA), Australian Group 1, 2, and 3 (identified in Australia), Italy02, and D274 (predominant IBV types identified in Europe, except 793B, Massachusetts, and LX4 types) have not to be tested, due to that these isolates are unavailable in our laboratory. However, the primers N (+) and N (−) could also be used to detect these IBV types, because the primers are targeting highly conserved regions among these IBV strains. It should be noted that although the primer targeting regions are conserved, N gene and 3′-terminal region of 3′ UTR show certain variations among different serotypes. It is likely that primers N (+) and N (−) may need slight modification to increase their universality for other IBV serotypes that have not been tested in our study. For example, degeneracy of primers should be considered which has been successfully applied in detection of viruses with genetic diversity.

5. We prepare homogenized tissue suspensions by using the TissueLyser II (Qiagen, Germany) which has been widely applied to sample preparation. The 2 ml microcentrifuge tubes with stainless steel beads for tissue disruption should be sterilized. Precooling the Tissue Lyser Adapter Set in −80 °C can reduce the RNA degradation in the process of sample preparation.

6. The repeated freeze-thaw cycles should facilitate viruses releasing from infected tissues. We aliquot the prepared samples (tissue and swab samples) into separate tubes, one tube for virus isolation and subsequent RNA extraction and the others kept at −80 °C for long-term storage.

7. Filtration of tissue and swab samples is not recommended because this step will reduce virus titer.

8. During the RNA extraction process, the most important preventative measure is to avoid RNA degradation caused by RNase contamination. All pipette tips and microcentrifuge tubes should be RNase-free and glove and mask should be worn.

9. The RNA pellet is often invisible and locates at the side and bottom of the tube. Discarding the supernatant should be performed carefully without touching the RNA pellet.

10. Do not allow the RNA to dry completely, which reduces the solubility of the RNA.

11. The one-step RT-PCR kit is employed to reduce the amount of handling required. In our laboratory, we have successfully used it to amplify RT-PCR products of between 1052 and 2849 bp in length from clinical samples.

12. General procedures to prevent PCR cross-contamination should be strictly followed. In order to prevent the detection of false positive, which may occur owing to cross-contamination, preparation of the master mix for RT-PCR should be carried out in an isolated room separate from areas used for sample processing and RNA extraction. If possible, each step of the whole process including sample processing, RT-PCR, and post-PCR analysis should be carried out in separated rooms.

13. To ensure the reliability of results, multiple positive and negative controls should be included in the RT-PCR reactions, especially when unknown clinical samples are tested. The negative control consists of a sample containing only the RT-PCR mix without RNA (2 μl of water is added instead of RNA). RNA of IBV (e.g., H120) can be used as positive control.

14. When adding the RNA samples to the RT-PCR mix, precaution must be taken to avoid RNA cross-contamination. Avoiding the formation of aerosols by using aerosol-resistant filtered pipette tips can prevent the false-positive results due to cross-sample contamination caused by aerosol spraying.

Acknowledgments

This work was supported by grants from the China Agriculture Research System (No. CARS-41-K12) and National "Twelfth Five-Year" Plan for Science & Technology Support (2015BAD12B03).

References

1. Cavanagh D (2007) Coronavirus avian infectious bronchitis virus. Vet Res 38:281–297

2. Han Z, Sun C, Yan B, Zhang X, Wang Y, Li C, Zhang Q, Ma Y, Shao Y, Liu Q (2011) A 15-year analysis of molecular epidemiology of avian infectious bronchitis coronavirus in China. Infect Genet Evol 11:190–200

3. Cavanagh D (2005) Coronaviruses in poultry and other birds. Avian Pathol 34:439–448

4. Cook JKA, Jackwood M, Jones R (2012) The long view: 40 years of infectious bronchitis research. Avian Pathol 41:239–250

5. Jackwood MW, Hall D, Handel A (2012) Molecular evolution and emergence of avian gammacoronaviruses. Infect Genet Evol 12:1305–1311

6. Sun C, Han Z, Ma H, Zhang Q, Yan B, Shao Y, Xu J, Kong X, Liu S (2011) Phylogenetic analysis of infectious bronchitis coronaviruses newly isolated in China, and pathogenicity and evaluation of protection induced by Massachusetts serotype H120 vaccine against QX-like strains. Avian Pathol 40:43–54

7. Ma H, Shao Y, Sun C, Han Z, Liu X, Guo H, Kong X, Liu S (2012) Genetic diversity of avian infectious bronchitis coronavirus in recent years in China. Avian Dis 56:15–28

8. Cavanagh D (2001) Innovation and discovery: the application of nucleic acid-based technology to avian virus detection and characterization. Avian Pathol 30:581–598

9. Cavanagh D, Mawditt K, Sharma M, Drury SE, Ainsworth HL, Britton P, Gough RE (2001) Detection of a coronavirus from turkey poults in Europe genetically related to infectious bronchitis virus of chickens. Avian Pathol 30:355–368

10. Jones R, Ellis R, Cox W, Errington J, Fuller C, Irvine R, Wakeley P (2011) Development and validation of RT-PCR tests for the detection and S1 genotyping of infectious bronchitis virus and other closely related gammacoronaviruses within clinical samples. Transbound Emerg Dis 58:411–420

11. Meir R, Maharat O, Farnushi Y, Simanov L (2010) Development of a real-time TaqMan(R) RT-PCR assay for the detection of infectious bronchitis virus in chickens, and comparison of RT-PCR and virus isolation. J Virol Methods 163:190–194

12. Callison SA, Hilt DA, Boynton TO, Sample BF, Robison R, Swayne DE, Jackwood MW (2006) Development and evaluation of a real-time Taqman RT-PCR assay for the detection of infectious bronchitis virus from infected chickens. J Virol Methods 138:60–65

13. Williams AK, Wang L, Sneed LW, Collisson EW (1992) Comparative analyses of the nucleocapsid genes of several strains of infectious bronchitis virus and other coronaviruses. Virus Res 25:213–222

14. Zhao X, Shaw K, Cavanagh D (1993) Presence of subgenomic mRNAs in virions of coronavirus IBV. Virology 196:172–178

15. Enjuanes L, Almazán F, Sola I, Zuiga S (2006) Biochemical aspects of coronavirus replication and virus-host interaction. Annu Rev Microbiol 60:211–230

16. Han Z, Zhao F, Shao Y, Liu X, Kong X, Song Y, Liu S (2013) Fine level epitope mapping and conservation analysis of two novel linear B-cell epitopes of the avian infectious bronchitis coronavirus nucleocapsid protein. Virus Res 171:54–64

Chapter 12

A Multiplex Polymerase Chain Reaction for Differential Detection of Turkey Coronavirus from Chicken Infectious Bronchitis Virus and Bovine Coronavirus

Chien Chang Loa, Ching Ching Wu, and Tsang Long Lin

Abstract

A multiplex polymerase chain reaction (PCR) method for differential detection of turkey coronavirus (TCoV), infectious bronchitis virus (IBV), and bovine coronavirus (BCoV) is presented in this chapter. Primers are designed from the conserved or variable regions of nucleocapsid (N) or spike (S) protein genes of TCoV, IBV, and BCoV and used in the same PCR reaction. Reverse transcription followed by PCR reaction is used to amplify a portion of N or S gene of the corresponding coronaviruses. Two PCR products, a 356-bp band corresponding to N gene and a 727-bp band corresponding to S gene, are obtained for TCoV. In contrast, one PCR product of 356 bp corresponding to a fragment of N gene is obtained for IBV strains and one PCR product of 568 bp corresponding to a fragment of S gene is obtained for BCoV.

Key words Multiplex PCR, Differential detection, Coronavirus, Nucleocapsid gene, Spike gene

1 Introduction

Turkey coronavirus (TCoV) contributed to significant economic losses and remains as a serious threat to the turkey producers. Turkey coronaviral enteritis in areas with high concentrations of turkeys on a year-round basis is not easily eliminated and is encountered frequently in turkey poults [1]. Accurate and rapid method for diagnosis of TCoV infection is the key to effective control of the disease.

Turkey coronavirus belongs to the family Coronaviridae, which is a group of enveloped, positive-stranded RNA viruses that infect a wide range of mammalian and avian species. The major structural proteins of coronavirus include phosphorylated nucleocapsid (N) protein, peplomeric spike (S) glycoprotein, and transmembrane or membrane (M) glycoprotein. Spike protein contributes to the distinctive peplomers on the viral surface and contains neutralizing and group-specific epitopes. Spike protein is highly variable among

Leyi Wang (ed.), *Animal Coronaviruses*, Springer Protocols Handbooks,
DOI 10.1007/978-1-4939-3414-0_12, © Springer Science+Business Media New York 2016

different coronaviruses while M and N proteins are more conserved among coronaviruses between different antigenic groups [2].

There is a close antigenic and genomic relationship between TCoV and infectious bronchitis virus (IBV) according to studies of immunofluorescent antibody assay (IFA), enzyme-linked immunosorbent assay (ELISA), and sequence analysis in our and other laboratories [3–8]. In addition, bovine coronavirus (BCoV) was demonstrated to cause experimental enteric infection in turkey [9]. Therefore, close relationship between TCoV and BCoV was previously reported and TCoV was placed in an antigenic group as BCoV [10, 11]. Although the sequence data revealed divergence of S genes among TCoV, IBV, and BCoV [12–14], there is still a need to detect and differentiate them accurately and quickly. Polymerase chain reaction (PCR) assay has been an important approach for detecting many veterinary important microorganisms with the distinct advantages of high sensitivity and specificity. This chapter describes a multiplex PCR assay to detect and differentiate TCoV, IBV, and BCoV in a single reaction [15].

2   Materials

2.1   Viral RNA Preparation

1. Test sample: Turkey intestine.
2. Phosphate-buffered saline (PBS), pH 7.4.
3. Stomacher® 80 microBiomaster laboratory paddle blenders (Seward, Davie, FL, USA).
4. RNApure reagent (GenHunter, Nashville, TN, USA).
5. Chloroform.
6. Isopropanol.
7. 70 % Ethanol.
8. Diethyl-pyrocarbonate (DEPC)-treated sterile double-distilled water (DEPC-H$_2$O).

2.2   Reverse Transcription

1. SuperScript III first-strand synthesis system for RT-PCR kit (Life Technologies/Invitrogen, Carlsbad, CA, USA).
2. RNaseOUT is a recombinant RNase inhibitor (Life Technologies/ Invitrogen).
3. Random hexamers (Life Technologies/Invitrogen).
4. Deoxynucleotide triphosphates (dNTP) (Promega Corp., Madison, WI, USA).

2.3   PCR Reaction

1. Primers listed in Table 1 (see Note 1).
2. Taq polymerase (Promega Corp).
3. Sterile distilled water.

Table 1
List of primers and sequences for coronavirus multiplex polymerase chain reaction

Name	Sequences
N103F	CCTGATGGTAATTTCCGTTGGG
N102R	ACGCCCATCCTTAATACCTTCCTC
S306F	TGTATCTAATTTGGGTGGGTTTGA
S306R	ATAAGCTGCTAATTGAAGGGATGC
S3	ATGTGTGTAGGTAATGGTCCTGG
S6	AGCAACTACGAATCATAAAA

4. PCR thermal cycler (GeneAmp PCR System 9600, Perkin Elmer Centers Corp., Norwalk, CT, USA).

5. Agarose.

6. Ethidium bromide, 0.5 µg/ml.

7. Ultraviolet transilluminator.

3 Methods

3.1 Viral RNA Preparation

1. Turkey intestines are cut into pieces and homogenized by Stomacher with fivefold volume of PBS solution.

2. The intestinal homogenates are clarified by centrifugation at $1500 \times g$ for 10 min. The supernatants containing TCoV are used as virus source for preparation of RNA templates for reverse transcription (RT)-PCR reaction.

3. Two hundred microliters of above supernatants are mixed with 1 ml of RNApure reagent and incubated on ice for 10 min (*see* **Note 2**).

4. Add 180 µl of chloroform, mix the mixture, and vortex vigorously for 10 s (*see* **Note 3**).

5. Centrifuge at $13,000 \times g$ for 10 min at 4 °C. Carefully take the upper aqueous phase into a clean tube and mix with equal volume of cold isopropanol by vortexing vigorously for 30 s. Incubate on ice for 10 min.

6. Centrifuge at $13,000 \times g$ for 10 min at 4 °C. Carefully discard the supernatant without disturbing RNA pellet.

7. Wash RNA pellet with 1 ml of cold 70 % ethanol. Incubate on ice for 5 min.

8. Centrifuge at $13,000 \times g$ for 2 min at 4 °C. Remove the ethanol. Spin briefly and remove the residual liquid with pipette (*see* **Note 4**).

9. Dissolve RNA pellet in 50 μl of DEPC-H_2O and a portion of it is quantified by spectrophotometry (GeneQuant Pro Spectrophotometer, Amersham Pharmacia Biotech, Inc., Piscataway, NJ, USA; GeneQuant 1300 Spectrophotometer, GE Healthcare Bio-Sciences, Piscataway, NJ, USA) at 260 nm wavelength (*see* **Note 5**).

10. Positive control samples including turkey intestinal homogenates containing TCoV/IN/540/94 (GenBank accession number EU022525), IBV strains (ATCC, Manassas, VA, USA), and BCoV (NVSL, Ames, IA, USA) are processed for viral RNA following the procedures above.

3.2 Reverse Transcription

1. Mix 8 μl (1 pg to 5 μg) of RNA with 1 μl (50 ng/μl) random hexamer and 1 μl (10 mM) dNTP in a total volume of 10 μl.

2. Incubate at 65 °C for 5 min and sit on ice for 1 min.

3. Add 10 μl of SuperScript III cDNA Synthesis Mix (containing 2 μl 10× RT buffer, 4 μl (25 mM) $MgCl_2$, 2 μl (0.1 M) DTT, 1 μl (40 U/μl) RNaseOUT, 1 μl (200 U/μl) SuperScript III RT enzyme) to each RNA/primer mixture.

4. Incubate at 25 °C for 10 min and followed by 50 °C for 50 min.

5. Terminate the RT reaction at 85 °C for 5 min and chill on ice (*see* **Note 6**).

3.3 PCR Reaction

1. Two microliters of cDNA are used in PCR amplifications. The components for 100 μl reaction mixture are listed in Table 2 (*see* **Note 7**).

2. PCR cyclic parameters: 94 °C for 30 s for denaturation, 50 °C for 1 min for annealing, 72 °C for 1 min for extension for 25 cycles followed by 72 °C for 10-min final extension.

3. A volume of 8 μl of the amplified PCR products is subjected to electrophoresis at 100 V in horizontal gels containing 1 % agarose. The gel is stained with ethidium bromide. Amplified DNA products are visualized by viewing the gel with an ultraviolet transilluminator, compared with standard markers of DNA size (*see* **Notes 8** and **9**).

4 Notes

1. Primers are based on the variable and conserved regions of S and N gene sequences among TCoV, IBV, and BCoV. The sense primer N103F and antisense primer N102R common to both TCoV and IBV were designed according to the conserved

Table 2
Preparation of reaction mixture for coronavirus multiplex polymerase chain reaction

Components	Volumes (μl)
Distilled H$_2$O	67
10× buffer	10
MgCl$_2$ (25 mM)	6
dNTP mix (10 mM)	2
Primer S3 (10 pmol/μl)	2
Primer S6 (10 pmol/μl)	2
Primer S306F (10 pmol/μl)	2
Primer S306R (10 pmol/μl)	2
Primer N103F (10 pmol/μl)	2
Primer N102R (10 pmol/μl)	2
Taq enzyme (5 U/μl)	1
cDNA template	2

regions of N gene sequences. This set of primers specified a 356-bp sequence corresponding to nucleotide position 445 to 801 of TCoV N gene. The sense primer S306F and antisense primer S306R specific to TCoV were designed according to the variable regions of S gene sequences among these viruses. This set of primers specified a 727-bp sequence corresponding to the nucleotide position 2019 to 2745 of TCoV S gene. The sense primer S3 and antisense primer S6 specific to BCoV were designed according to the variable regions of S gene sequences among these viruses. This set of primers specified a 568-bp sequence corresponding to the nucleotide position 1488 to 2055 of BCoV S gene.

2. The suggested ratio of RNApure reagent to sample is 10:1. Excess amount of RNApure reagent has no negative impact. The lower ratio (5:1) in this step is intended to obtain higher concentration of viral RNA in the final supernatants. If the upper aqueous phase after centrifugation at step 5 is more than half of the total volume, there is not enough RNApure reagent added. The appropriate reagent amount may be adjusted. Chloroform is applied at 150 μl for every ml of lysate.

3. The sample mixture with chloroform at this step can be stored at −70 °C or lower than −70 °C before proceeding to the next step.

4. Optional: Invert the tube for 5–10 min for air-drying of RNA pellet is a helpful tip to completely remove any residual ethanol that may interfere with the following RT reaction.

5. It is critical to make sure that the jellylike RNA pellet is completely dissolved into solution by repeat pipetting. The volume (50 μl) of DEPC-H$_2$O may be adjusted according to RNA pellet size for appropriate RNA concentration. Concentration can be estimated by taking 1 μl of the RNA solution into 1 ml of water. Read at 260 nm. 1 OD260 = 40 μg. The RNA quality can be further examined by OD 260/280 and 260/230 ratio. The ratio of 260/280 about 2.0 is considered as pure for RNA, while 1.8 is considered pure for DNA. The expected 260/230 ratio is around 2.0 to 2.2 for pure nucleic acid. If the ratio is appreciably lower, it may indicate the presence of protein, phenol, or other contaminants with strong absorption near 280 or 230 nm. RNA should be stored at −70 °C or lower than −70 °C.

6. The synthesized cDNA in the RT reaction can be stored at −20 °C or lower than −20 °C until used. RNase H digestion to remove the RNA templates from the cDNA:RNA hybrid molecule is optional. The RNase treatment may increase PCR sensitivity for long templates. The target products (356, 568, and 727 bp) of this multiplex PCR are not considered long. The benefit of this RNase digestion is likely limited.

7. For routine practice in the laboratory for large number of samples, 25 μl reaction can be applied with reduced cost of reagents.

8. Result interpretation:

   TCoV positive: two PCR products, a 356-bp band, and a 727-bp band.

   IBV positive: one PCR product of 356 bp.

   BCoV positive: one PCR product of 568 bp.

   Negative: no PCR product.

   One limitation of this multiplex PCR should be noted. When both TCoV and IBV are present in the sample, the IBV-positive PCR product at 356 bp is overlapping with one of the two TCoV PCR products. The result of two PCR product bands at 356 and 727 bp reflects a confirmed diagnosis of TCoV positive but does not rule out the presence of IBV. This concern is alleviated by tissue tropism of IBV. Turkey enteric infection by chicken respiratory IBV has never been reported. Accordingly, the presence of IBV in turkey intestines (the test sample) is not likely. Any such concern should be further evaluated by a separate PCR specific for IBV [16]. On the other hand, IBV-positive result is able to exclude the presence of TCoV.

9. The sensitivity of this multiplex PCR is 4.8×10^{-3} μg of TCoV RNA, 4.6×10^{-4} μg of IBV RNA, and 8.0×10^{-2} μg of BCoV RNA. The specificity had been evaluated against Newcastle disease virus, Marek's disease virus, turkey pox virus, pigeon pox virus, fowl pox virus, reovirus, infectious bursal disease virus, enterovirus, astrovirus, *Salmonella enterica*, *Escherichia coli*, and *Mycoplasma gallisepticum* with negative results that have no PCR products.

Acknowledgements

The protocol "A multiplex polymerase chain reaction for differential detection of turkey coronavirus from chicken infectious bronchitis virus and bovine coronavirus" outlined in this chapter had been successfully carried out in the authors' studies on molecular diagnostics and molecular virology of turkey coronavirus infection in turkeys. Those studies were in part financially supported by USDA, North Carolina Poultry Federation, and/or Indiana Department of Agriculture and technically assisted by Drs. Tom Brien and David Hermes, Mr. Tom Hooper, and Ms. Donna Schrader for clinical and diagnostic investigation, virus isolation and propagation, and animal experimentation.

References

1. Nagaraja KV, Pomeroy BS (1997) Coronaviral enteritis of turkeys (blue comb disease). In: Calnek BW, Barnes HJ, Beard CW et al (eds) Diseases of poultry, 10th edn. Iowa state University Press, Ames, IA

2. Saif LJ (1993) Coronavirus immunogens. Vet Microbiol 37:285–297

3. Guy JS, Barnes HJ, Smith LG, Breslin J (1997) Antigenic characterization of a turkey coronavirus identified in poult enteritis and mortality syndrome-affected turkeys. Avian Dis 41:583–590

4. Stephensen CB, Casebolt DB, Gangopadhyay NN (1999) Phylogenetic analysis of a highly conserved region of the polymerase gene from 11 coronaviruses and development of a consensus polymerase chain reaction assay. Virus Res 60:181–189

5. Breslin JJ, Smith LG, Fuller FJ, Guy JS (1999) Sequence analysis of the matrix/nucleocapsid gene region of turkey coronavirus. Intervirology 42:22–29

6. Breslin JJ, Smith LG, Fuller FJ, Guy JS (1999) Sequence analysis of the turkey coronavirus nucleocapsid protein gene and 3' untranslated region identifies the virus as a close relative of infectious bronchitis virus. Virus Res 65:187–193

7. Loa CC, Lin TL, Wu CC, Bryan TA, Thacker HL, Hooper T, Schrader D (2000) Detection of antibody to turkey coronavirus by antibody-capture enzyme-linked immunosorbent assay utilizing infectious bronchitis virus antigen. Avian Dis 44:498–506

8. Akin A, Lin TL, Wu CC, Bryan TA, Hooper T, Schrader D (2001) Nucleocapsid protein gene sequence analysis reveals close genomic relationship between turkey coronavirus and avian infectious bronchitis virus. Acta Virol 45(1):31–38

9. Ismail MM, Cho KO, Ward LA, Saif LJ, Saif YM (2001) Experimental bovine coronavirus in turkey poults and young chickens. Avian Dis 45:157–163

10. Dea S, Verbeek AJ, Tijssen P (1990) Antigenic and genomic relationships among turkey and bovine enteric coronaviruses. J Virol 64:3112–3118

11. Verbeek A, Tijssen P (1991) Sequence analysis of the turkey enteric coronavirus nucleocapsid and membrane protein genes: a close genomic relationship with bovine coronavirus. J Gen Virol 72:1659–1666

12. Lin TL, Loa CC, Wu CC (2004) Complete sequences of 3′end coding region for structural protein genes of turkey coronavirus. Virus Res 106(1):61–70

13. Loa CC, Lin TL, Wu CC, Bryan TA, Hooper T, Schrader D (2006) Comparison of 3′ end encoding regions of turkey coronavirus isolates from Indiana, North Carolina, and Minnesota. Intervirology 49(4):230–238

14. Cao J, Wu CC, Lin TL (2008) Complete nucleotide sequence of polyprotein gene 1 and genome organization of turkey coronavirus. Virus Res 136(1-2):43–49

15. Loa CC, Lin TL, Wu CC, Bryan TA, Hooper T, Schrader D (2006) Differential detection of turkey coronavirus, infectious bronchitis virus, and bovine coronavirus by a multiplex polymerase chain reaction. J Virol Methods 131:86–91

16. Lee CW, Hilt DA, Jackwood MW (2000) Redesign of primers and application of the reverse transcriptase-polymerase chain reaction and restriction fragment length polymorphism test to the DE072 strain of infectious bronchitis virus. Avian Dis 44:650–654

Chapter 13

Real-Time Reverse Transcription-Polymerase Chain Reaction for Detection and Quantitation of Turkey Coronavirus RNA in Feces and Intestine Tissues

Yi-Ning Chen, Ching Ching Wu, and Tsang Long Lin

Abstract

Turkey coronavirus (TCoV) infection causes acute atrophic enteritis in turkey poults, leading to significant economic loss in the turkey industry. Rapid detection, differentiation, and quantitation of TCoV are critical to the diagnosis and control of the disease. A specific one-step real-time reverse transcription-polymerase chain reaction (RT-PCR) assay using TCoV-specific primers and dual-labeled fluorescent probe for detection and quantitation of TCoV in feces and intestine tissues is described in this chapter. The fluorogenic probe labeled with a reporter dye (FAM, 6-carboxytetramethylrhodamine) and a quencher dye (Absolute Quencher™) was designed to bind to a 186 base-pair fragment flanked by the two PCR primers targeting the 3′ end of spike gene (S2) of TCoV. The assay is highly specific and sensitive and can quantitate between 10^2 and 10^{10} copies/mL of viral genome. It is useful in monitoring the progression of TCoV-induced atrophic enteritis in the turkey flocks.

Key words Turkey coronavirus, Real-time RT-PCR, TaqMan probe, Spike gene, Intestine, Feces

1 Introduction

Turkey coronavirus (TCoV) causes atrophic enteritis in turkeys and outbreaks or cases of turkey coronaviral enteritis occurred and still occurs in the USA [1], Canada [2], Brazil [3], and Europe [4]. TCoV belongs to species *Avian coronavirus* of the genus *Gammacoronavirus* in the family *Coronaviridae*. The genome of TCoV is a linear positive-sense single-stranded RNA encoding three major structural proteins including spike (S), membrane (M), and nucleocapsid (N) protein. The amino terminal region of S protein (S1) containing receptor-binding domain and neutralizing epitopes can determine host specificity and induce the production of neutralizing antibodies [5]. The carboxyl terminal region of S protein (S2) consisting of transmembrane domain is responsible for cell fusion and virus assembly [6]. S gene is a more common target used for coronavirus (CoV) differentiation because S gene is

Leyi Wang (ed.), *Animal Coronaviruses*, Springer Protocols Handbooks,
DOI 10.1007/978-1-4939-3414-0_13, © Springer Science+Business Media New York 2016

highly variable among different CoVs while M and N genes are more conserved. Within the S gene, the S2 gene is more conserved than S1 gene between different CoVs and between different isolates or strains of the same CoV [7]. Therefore, S2 gene is chosen as a target to detect TCoV and differentiate TCoV from other CoVs.

There is no cell culture system for TCoV; thus virus isolation is not feasible. Because the sequence information of TCoV is available, reverse transcription-polymerase chain reaction (RT-PCR)-based methods with high specificity and sensitivity have been developed [7, 8]. Real-time RT-PCR illustrated here uses a pair of TCoV-specific primers targeting a 186 base-pair fragment of TCoV S2 gene and a dual-labeled probe with a reporter dye (FAM) and a quencher dye (Absolute Quencher™) combined with the 5′ to 3′ exonuclease activity of *Taq* polymerase to increase the release of reporter dye fluorescence in the course of PCR amplification [9]. Quantitative data can be accessed by the standard curve established with serial dilutions of standard RNA. The procedure does not need post-PCR electrophoresis, so the processing time can be significantly reduced and the risks for carryover and cross-contamination between samples can be lessened. In this chapter, the protocol for one-step real-time RT-PCR to detect, differentiate, and quantitative TCoV RNA in the feces and intestinal tissue is presented. In **step** 1, feces or intestine tissues were collected into RNA*later* RNA stabilization reagent. In **step** 2, TCoV RNA was extracted from feces using QIAamp viral RNA mini kit or intestine tissues using RNAeasy mini kit. In **step** 3, the extracted RNA was subjected to one-step real-time RT-PCR for detection and quantitation of TCoV in feces or intestine tissues. In **step** 4, a standard curve was established by serially diluted in vitro-transcribed RNA for absolute quantitation of TCoV.

2 Materials

2.1 Sample Collection

2.1.1 Reagents

1. Diethyl pyrocarbonate (DEPC) (Sigma-Aldrich, St. Louis, MO, USA): DEPC is very sensitive to moisture, so it needs to be stored at 2–8 °C to help reduce exposure to moisture.

2. Preparation of DEPC-treated water (DEPC-H₂O):

   (a) Prepare 0.1 % (v/v) DEPC in the water undergone reverse osmosis filtration and deionization. Add 0.1 mL DEPC solution to 100 mL of water. DEPC appears as globules and needs continuous stirring until the globules disappear. It takes 12 h at 37 °C in a fume hood. DEPC can dissolve plastic, so it is better to store DEPC solution in a glass bottle.

(b) Autoclave 0.1 % DEPC solution at 121 °C for 15 min to remove any trace of DEPC. The autoclaved DEPC-H$_2$O can be stored at any temperature.

3. RNA*later* RNA stabilization solution (Qiagen, Valencia, CA, USA): It can be stored at room temperature (15–25 °C) for at least 1 year. Samples in RNAlater stabilization reagent can be kept at 37 °C for 1 day, 15–25 °C (room temperature) for 7 days, 2–8 °C (refrigerator) for 4 weeks, and –20 or –80 °C for a longer storage. Samples in RNAlater stabilization reagent stored at –20 or –80 °C can remain stable for 20 rounds of freeze and thaw.

4. β-Mercaptoethanol (Sigma-Aldrich, St. Louis, MO, USA): It should be stored at 2–8 °C and processed in a chemical hood.

5. Phosphate-buffered saline (PBS) is composed of 1.44 g Na$_2$HPO$_4$, 8 g NaCl, 0.24 g KH$_2$PO$_4$, and 0.2 g KCl in 1 L ddH$_2$O. The solution is adjusted to pH 7.2 and autoclaved before use.

2.2 RNA Extraction

2.2.1 Reagents

1. RNase AWAY™ spray (VWR, Batavia, IL, USA): It is a surfactant that removes RNA and RNases from laboratory equipment and glassware.

2. Absolute ethanol (200 Proof) (Thermo Fisher Scientific, Waltham, MA, USA): ≥99.5 % (v/v), molecular biology grade, DNase-, RNase-, and protease-free.

3. QIAamp® viral RNA mini kit (Qiagen, Valencia, CA, USA): The kit contains lyophilized carrier RNA, Buffer AVL (lysis), AW1 (wash), AW2 (wash), and AVE (elute). Buffer AVL and AW1 contain guanidine thiocyanate, which is hazardous to health. Viral RNA can bind specifically to the silica membrane of QIAamp spin columns and pure viral RNA is eluted in either water or Buffer AVE.

(a) Prepare carrier RNA: Add 310 μL Buffer AVE to the tube containing 310 μg lyophilized carrier RNA to obtain a solution of 1 μg/μL and store it at –20 °C. Do not freeze–thaw the aliquots of carrier RNA more than three times. Incubate Buffer AVL at 80 °C if it has precipitate until it is dissolved. Add 100 volumes of Buffer AVL to 1 volume of carrier RNA-AVE solution. Mix gently by inverting tubes ten times without using a vortexer to avoid any foaming. AVL-carrier RNA solution can be stored at 4 °C for 48 h. Incubate AVL-carrier RNA solution at 80 °C for less than 5 min if there is precipitant. Do not warm the solution more than six times.

(b) Add 25 mL of 96–100 % ethanol into 19 mL of concentrated Buffer AW1.

(c) Add 30 mL of 96–100 % ethanol into 13 mL of concentrated Buffer AW2.

4. RNeasy mini kit (Qiagen, Valencia, CA, USA): The kit contains Buffer RLT (lysis), RW1 (wash), and RPE (elute). Buffer RLT and AW1 contain guanidine thiocyanate, which is harmful. RNA from intestine tissues can bind to silica membrane of RNeasy spin columns with a binding capacity of 100 µg.

(a) Add 10 µL β-mercaptoethanol (β-ME) per 1 mL Buffer RLT in a fume hood. Buffer BLT with β-ME can be stored at room temperature for up to 1 month.

(b) Add 44 mL of 96–100 % ethanol to 11 mL of concentrated Buffer RPE.

2.2.2 Equipment

1. Bio-Gen Pro200 homogenizer (Pro Scientific, Oxford, CT, USA).

2. GeneQuant 1300 Spectrophotometer (GE Healthcare Bio-Sciences, Piscataway, NJ, USA).

3. Eppendorf 5424 Centrifuge (Eppendorf, Hamburg, Germany).

2.3 Real-Time RT-PCR

2.3.1 Reagent

1. Primers and probe can be synthesized by Integrated DNA Technologies (IDT, San Jose, CA, USA). The primers and primer sequence information are listed in Table 1. The lyophilized powders of products prepared by company are to be dissolved in DEPC-H_2O to 100 µM as stock solution (100×). The working solution of primers and probe is 10 µM. Both stock and working solution of primers and probe are stored at –20 °C.

2. Platinum® Quantitative RT-PCR ThermoScript™ One-Step System (Invitrogen™, Life Technologies, Grand Island, NY, USA): It can be stored at –20 °C for at least 6 months. The kit contains ThermoScript™ RT/Platinum® *Taq* mix, 2× ThermoScript™ reaction mix (a buffer containing 0.4 mM of each dNTP, 6 mM $MgSO_4$), and a vial of 50 mM $MgSO_4$.

2.3.2 Equipment

1. Rotor-Gene 3000™ real-time thermocycler (Corbett Research, Sydney, Australia): This model was discontinued. The alternative model is Rotor-Gene Q provided by Qiagen (Valencia, CA, USA).

Table 1
Primers and sequence information for turkey coronavirus real-time RT-PCR

Primer	5′ → 3′ sequence
QS1F	TCGCAATCTATGCGATATG
QS1R	CAGTCTTGGGCATTACAC
QS1P	Absolute Quencher-TCTGTGGCAATGGTAGCCATGTTC-FAM
6F	GACCATGGGATTTGTTGAA
6R	TTTTTAATGGCATCTTTTGA

2.4 Standard Curve	

2.4 Standard Curve

2.4.1 Reagent

1. pTriEx™-3 DNA-Novagen vector (EMD Millipore Corporation, Billerica, MA, USA): The vector was sold by Novagen (Madison, WI, USA) originally and is handled by Merck Millipore now. The availability of this vector is limited. Alternatively, any vector using T7 promotor can be used for in vitro transcription in the current protocol.

2. Restriction enzymes, *Kpn*I and *Nco*I (New England Bio Labs Inc., Ipswich, MA, USA).

3. T4 DNA ligase (Promega, Madison, WI, USA).

4. QIAprep Spin Miniprep kit (Qiagen, Valencia, CA, USA).

5. RiboMAX™ large-scale RNA production system-T7 (Promega, Madison, WI, USA): The kit contains enzyme (RNA Polymerase, Recombinant RNasin® Ribonuclease Inhibitor and Recombinant Inorganic Pyrophosphatase), transcription 5× buffer, each of 4rNTPs (100 mM), RQ1 RNase-free DNase (1 U/μL), 3 M sodium acetate (pH 5.2), and nuclease-free water.

6. RQ1 DNase (Promega, Madison, WI, USA).

7. DNA clean and concentration™-5 kit (Zymo, Irvine, CA, USA): The kit contains DNA-binding buffer, Zymo-Spin™ Column, DNA wash buffer, and DNA elution buffer.

3 Methods

3.1 Sample Collection

3.1.1 Feces from Cloaca of Turkeys

1. Use individual packed sterile cotton swab to take feces from turkey cloaca.

2. Place about 100 mg of feces on the swab into a 1.7 mL microcentrifuge tube containing 1 mL of RNA*later* RNA stabilization reagent. The space occupied by 100 mg feces is about 1/3 to 1/4 of 1.7 mL microcentrifuge tube.

3. Use sterile tips to suspend fecal matters in RNA*later* RNA stabilization reagent (*see* **Note 1**).

3.1.2 Feces from Floor

1. Use sterile forceps rinsed with DEPC-H_2O to collect fresh feces from floor and place about 100 mg of feces into a 1.7 mL microcentrifuge tube containing 1 mL of RNA*later* RNA stabilization reagent. The space occupied by 100 mg feces is about 1/3 to 1/4 of 1.7 mL microcentrifuge tube.

2. Use sterile tips to suspend fecal matters in RNA*later* RNA stabilization reagent (*see* **Note 1**).

3.1.3 Intestine Tissue

1. Use sterile forceps and scissors to cut 0.5 cm long segment of duodenum, jejunum, ileum, or cecum.

2. Use the scissors to open the intestine segment longitudinally and rinse away intestinal content with chill sterile phosphate-buffered saline (PBS, pH = 7.2).

3. Put the rinsed intestine segment into a 1.7 mL microcentrifuge tube containing 1 mL of RNA*later* RNA stabilization reagent (*see* **Note 2**).

3.2 RNA Extraction

3.2.1 Fecal Samples Using QIAamp® Viral RNA Mini Kit

1. Take 1.7 mL microcentrifuge tubes containing feces and RNA*later* RNA stabilization reagent for centrifugation at 3 3000 rpm (845 × *g*) for 2 min at 4 °C.

2. Take 140 μL of supernatant into 560 μL of prepared Buffer AVL containing carrier RNA in a 1.7 mL microcentrifuge tube.

3. Incubate at room temperature for 10 min.

4. Briefly centrifuge the tube to remove drops from the inside of the lid.

5. Add 560 μL of 96–100 % ethanol to the sample and mix by pulse-vortexing for 15 s. After mixing, briefly centrifuge the tube to remove drops from the inside of the lid.

6. Apply 630 μL of the solution from **step** 5 to the QIAamp spin column in a 2 mL collection tube and centrifuge at 8000 rpm (6010 × *g*) for 1 min. Discard the old 2 mL tube containing the filtrate and transfer the QIAamp spin column to a new 2 mL collection tube.

7. Apply remaining part of the solution from **step** 5 to the QIAamp spin column and centrifuge at 8000 rpm for 1 min. Discard the old 2 mL containing the filtrate and transfer the QIAamp spin column to another new 2 mL collection tube.

8. Add 500 μL of Buffer AW1 and centrifuge at 8000 rpm for 1 min. Place the QIAamp spin column into a clean 2 mL collection tube and discard the tube containing the filtrate.

9. Add 500 μL of Buffer AW2 and centrifuge at 14,000 rpm (18407 × *g*) for 3 min. Change the direction of tubes and centrifuge at 14,000 rpm for another 1 min.

10. Place the QIAamp spin column in a clean 1.7 mL microcentrifuge tube and add 60 μL of Buffer AVE. Incubate at room temperature for 1 min and centrifuge at 8000 rpm for 1 min.

11. Take 4 μL RNA into 96 μL Buffer AVE and measure the amount of RNA by GeneQuant following the manufacturer's instruction.

12. Aliquot the RNA into 5 μL each tube and store in −80 °C freezer for use in real-time RT-PCR.

3.2.2 Intestine Tissue Samples Using RNeasy Mini Kit

1. Take intestine segment out of 1.7 mL microcentrifuge tubes containing 1 mL of RNA*later* RNA stabilization reagent and put the tissue specimen on top of the plastic paper treated with RNase Away and DEPC H$_2$O.

2. Use sterile forceps and scissors to cut the tissue into small pieces at room temperature.

3. Weight 30 mg of tissue and homogenize it in 600 μL of Buffer RLT by using Pro200 homogenizer (*see* **Note 3**).

4. Centrifuge the lysate from **step** 3 at 14,000 rpm for 3 min. Transfer the supernatant to a new 1.7 mL tube.

5. Add the same volume of 70 % ethanol to the supernatant and mix immediately by pipetting. Transfer 700 μL of the mixture to the RNeasy spin column in a 2 mL collection tube.

6. Centrifuge at 10,000 rpm (9391 × *g*) for 15 s. Discard the filtrate inside the 2 mL collection tube and place the same 2 mL collection tube back with the RNeasy spin column.

7. Apply the remaining part of mixture in **step** 5 to the same RNeasy spin column and centrifuge at 10,000 rpm for 15 s. Discard the filtrate inside the 2 mL collection tube and place the same 2 mL collection tube back with the RNeasy spin column.

8. Add 700 μL Buffer RW1 to the RNeasy spin column and centrifuge at 10,000 rpm for 15 s. Discard the filtrate and reuse the 2 mL collection tube.

9. Add 500 μL Buffer RPE to the RNeasy spin column and centrifuge at 10,000 rpm for 15 s. Discard the filtrate and reuse the 2 mL collection tube.

10. Add another 500 μL Buffer RPE to the RNeasy spin column and centrifuge at 10,000 rpm for 15 s.

11. Place the RNeasy spin column into a new 2 mL collection tube. Discard the 2 mL collection tube containing the filtrate. Centrifuge at 14,000 rpm for 1 min to get rid of the remaining ethanol.

12. Place the RNeasy spin column into a 1.7 mL microcentrifuge tube. Add 50 μL of DEPC-H_2O and centrifuge at 10,000 rpm for 1 min to elute RNA.

13. Take 4 μL RNA into 96 μL DEPC-H_2O and measure the amount of RNA by GeneQuant 1300. If the RNA yield is higher than 30 μg (0.6 μg/μL), repeat the elution step to recover the remaining RNA inside the RNeasy spin column.

14. Aliquot the RNA into 5 μL tube individually and store in −80 °C freezer for use in real-time RT-PCR.

3.3 One-Step Real-Time RT-PCR

1. Prepare a total of 25 μL of reaction mixture (Table 2) on ice by using TCoV-specific primers, probe, reaction buffer from Platinum® Quantitative RT-PCR ThermoScript™ One-Step System, and 5 μL of RNA template. Mix gently by pipetting up and down (*see* **Note 4**).

Table 2
Reaction mixture for one-step turkey coronavirus real-time RT-PCR

Components	Volume
RNA	5 μL
2× Reaction mix	12.5 μL
SuperScript™ III RT/platinum *Taq* Mix forward primer	0.5 μL
QS1F 10 μM	2.25 μL (900 nM)
Reverse primer QS1R 10 μM	0.75 μL (300 nM)
Probe QS1P 10 μM	0.5 μL (200 nM)
DEPC-H_2O	3.5 μL
Total volume	25 μL

2. Set up the following real-time RT-PCR conditions in Rotor-Gene 3000 or Rotor-Gene Q. The temperature profile is 50 °C for 30 min, 94 °C for 5 min, and 45 cycles of 94 °C for 20 s and 61 °C for 1 min to acquire the fluorescence FAM.

3. Every run of real-time RT-PCR should contain triple reactions for 9 standard concentrations of standard pTriEx3-6F/6R in vitro transcripts, non-template control (water), and samples.

4. Signals are regarded as positive if the fluorescence intensity exceeded ten times the standard deviation of the baseline fluorescence.

5. Calculate the concentration (copies/μL) of sample by blotting Ct values against the standard curve established by serial dilutions of TCoV standard transcripts from 10^2 to 10^{10} copies/μL in Sect. 3.4, **step 7** (*see* **Note 5**).

3.4 Standard Curve

1. Amplify partial S2 gene of TCoV in the region encompassing the fragment targeted by real-time RT-PCR by PCR with forward primer 6F and reverse primer 6R (Table 1) and the amplified fragment is designed as 6F/6R fragment. The fragments underlined in primers 6F and 6R are recognized by restriction enzymes *Nco*I and *Kpn*I, respectively.

2. Double-digest the pTriEx-3 DNA-Novagen (1–3 μg total) or 6F/6R fragment (1–3 μg total) with 1 μL of 1/10 diluted *Nco*I and 1 μL of 1/10 diluted *Kpn*I (NEB) in 50 μL reaction containing 5 μL of 10× NEB® Buffer 1 and 5 μL of bovine serum albumin (BSA, 1 mg/mL). Incubate the reaction at 37 °C for 1 h.

3. Ligate the treated pTriEx-3 and 6 F/6R fragment (638 bp) using T4 DNA ligase in 20 μL reaction to become pTriEx3-6F/6R. The reaction solution contains total 64 ng of the

prepared 6F/6R fragment (x μL), 2 μL of the prepared pTriEx vector (50 ng/μL), 2 μL 10× ligase buffer, 2 μL of 100 mM DTT, 1 μL of 10 mM ATP, 1 μL of T4 DNA ligase (0.2–0.4 Weiss units/μL), and nuclease-free water ($12 - x$ μL). Incubate the reaction at 16 °C for 2 h.

4. Generate in vitro transcripts of pTriEx3-6F/6R by using RiboMAX™ large-scale RNA production system-T7. Digest pTriEx3-6F/6R with restriction enzyme *NcoI* to linearize DNA template. Clean up the linearized DNA template with QIAprep Spin Miniprep kit (Qiagen). Prepare 100 μL reaction solution containing total 5–10 μg of linearized pTriEx-6F/6R (x μL), 20 μL of 5× T7 transcription buffer, 10 μL of T7 enzyme mix, 30 μL of rNTPs (25 mM ATP, CTP, GTP, UTP), and nuclease-free water ($40 - x$ μL). Incubate the reaction at 37 °C for 4 h to generate RNA transcript of pTriEx3-6F/6R.

5. Treat pTriEx3-6F/6R transcripts with RQ1 DNase (1 U/1 μg RNA, Promega), purify it by RNeasy mini kit, and measure the concentration of RNA by GeneQuant at 260 nm.

6. Make tenfold serial dilutions in DEPC-H_2O for real-time RT-PCR.

7. Create the standard curves by plotting the Ct value against each dilution of known concentration.

8. Calculate the copy number per micro liter by using the formula as follows:

$$\text{Copies} / \mu L = \left(ng / \mu L \times 10^9\right) / \left(MW \text{ of transcripts}\right) \times \left(6.023 \times 10^{23}\right).$$

4 Notes

1. RNAlater stabilization reagent is not designed for fecal samples but the previous study [10] showed a good stability of viral RNA in turkey feces by using RNAlater reagent. It is very critical to mix feces or cloacal swab with RNAlater to make feces submerged and contact RNAlater reagent completely for the stability of RNA in feces.

2. The thickness of tissue must be less than 0.5 cm. RNA in harvested intestine tissue is not protected until the tissue is completely submerged in a sufficient volume of RNAlater RNA Stabilization Reagent at about 10 μL reagent per 1 mg tissue. The intestinal content may interfere with the reaction of RNAlater reagent, so it is critical to wash off the intestinal contents. Insufficient RNA reagent may cause RNA degradation during storage. It is not recommended to harvest tissues frozen in liquid nitrogen or dry ice and later thaw them for RNAlater storage or RNA extraction because the process would cause severe RNA degradation.

3. The heat produced by the process of hominization can damage the integrity of RNA in intestine tissues leading to low sensitivity of real-time RT-PCR. Therefore, it is recommended to homogenize the intestine tissue for 30 s and cool the tube in ice in cycles until the intestine tissue is homogenized thoroughly.

4. Real-time RT-PCR is a very sensitive assay, so it is very easy to be interfered by bubbles created by pipetting. To use pipettes and take small volume of reagents (<10 μL) precisely, it is recommended to practice before performing the real test. In addition, the nonspecific reactions can be minimized by mixing reagents on the precooled (store at −20 °C freezer) aluminum loading block (Qiagen) on ice.

5. Example of running a set of samples from the setup to the end of calculating the copy number is illustrated below. First, collect ileum and cecum samples in RNAlater solution from three turkeys at 5 days post-infection of TCoV and the same kind of samples from negative control turkeys without TCoV infection. Second, label the samples from turkeys infected with TCoV as d5-i1 to d5-i3 and d5-c1to d5-c3, and those from negative control turkeys without TCoV infection as N-i1 to N-i3 and N-c1 to N-c3. Third, extract RNA from the samples according to Sect. 3.2.2. Next, arrange the samples in 96-well plate for one-step real-time RT-PCR (Table 3) and set up the real-time RT-PCR conditions. Prepare nuclease-free water as template for the non-template control

Table 3
Example of one-step real-time PCR: Sample arrangement in 96-well plate

	1	2	3	4	5	6	7	8	9
A	STD1	STD1	STD1	STD9	STD9	STD9	N-i2	N-i2	N-i2
B	STD2	STD2	STD2	d5-i1	d5-i1	d5-i1	N-i3	N-i3	N-i3
C	STD3	STD3	STD3	d5-i2	d5-i2	d5-i2	N-c1	N-c1	N-c1
D	STD4	STD4	STD4	d5-i3	d5-i3	d5-i3	N-c2	N-c2	N-c2
E	STD5	STD5	STD5	d5-c1	d5-c1	d5-c1	N-c3	N-c3	N-c3
F	STD6	STD6	STD6	d5-c2	d5-c2	d5-c2	NTC	NTC	NTC
G	STD7	STD7	STD7	d5-c3	d5-c3	d5-c3			
H	STD8	STD8	STD8	N-i1	N-i1	N-i1			

Samples are arranged in Row A to H from Column 1 to 12 in one 96-well plate. STD1 to STD8 are tenfold serially diluted standard RNA of pTriEx3-6F/6R from 10^2 to 10^9 copies/μL. NTC is nuclease-free water as template for real-time RT-PCR

(NTC) and tenfold serially diluted standard RNA of pTriEx3-6F/6R from 10^2 to 10^9 copies/μL, as STD1 to STD8. After the reaction complete, establish the standard curve formula based on the Ct values of STD1 to STD8. Then, calculate the copy numbers of the tested samples by the standard curve formula. Example for calculating sample concentration is illustrated in Table 4.

Table 4
Example of one-step real-time PCR: Ct values and copy numbers after calculation

Well ID	Sample	Ave Ct value	Ave Log 10 copies/μL	Ave copies/μL
A1-A3	STD1	40	2	100
B1-B3	STD2	37	3	1000
C1-C3	STD3	33	4	10,000
D1-D3	STD4	30	5	100,000
E1-E3	STD5	26	6	1,000,000
F1-E8	STD6	23	7	10,000,000
G1-G3	STD7	20	8	100,000,000
H1-H3	STD8	16	9	1,000,000,000
A4-A6	STD9	13	10	10,000,000,000
B4-B6	d5-i1	25	6.42	2,658,924
C4-C6	d5-i2	24	6.72	5,233,877
D4-D6	d5-i3	22	7.31	20,279,574
E4-E6	d5-c1	31	4.66	45,709
F4-F6	d5-c2	32	4.37	23,221
G4-G6	d5-c3	35	3.48	3045
H4-H6	N-i1	Over 45		UDL
A7-A9	N-i2	Over 45		UDL
B7-B9	N-i3	Over 45		UDL
C7-C9	N-c1	Over 45		UDL
D7-D9	N-c2	Over 45		UDL
E7-E9	N-c3	Over 45		UDL
F7-F9	NTC	Over 45		UDL

The standard curve formula is established by the Ct values and the copy numbers (Log 10 copies/μL) of STD1 to STD8: $Y = -3.4167X + 46.917$ ($R^2 = 0.9988$). Y is Ct value acquired by real-time RT-PCR and X is sample concentration presented by copies/μL. UDL is under detection limit

Acknowledgement

The protocol "Real-time reverse transcription-polymerase chain reaction for detection and quantitation of turkey coronavirus RNA in feces and intestine tissues" outlined in this chapter had been successfully carried out in the authors' studies on molecular diagnostics, molecular virology, immunology, and/or vaccinology of turkey coronaviral enteritis. Those studies were in part financially supported by USDA, North Carolina Poultry Federation, and/or Indiana Department of Agriculture and technically assisted by Drs. Tom Brien and David Hermes, Mr. Tom Hooper, and Ms. Donna Schrader for clinical investigation, virus isolation and propagation, and animal experimentation.

References

1. Day JM, Gonder E, Jennings S et al (2014) Investigating turkey enteric coronavirus circulating in the Southeastern United States and Arkansas during 2012 and 2013. Avian Dis 58:313–317

2. Gomaa MH, Yoo D, Ojkic D et al (2009) Infection with a pathogenic turkey coronavirus isolate negatively affects growth performance and intestinal morphology of young turkey poults in Canada. Avian Pathol 38:279–286

3. Teixeira MC, Luvizotto MC, Ferrari HF et al (2007) Detection of turkey coronavirus in commercial turkey poults in Brazil. Avian Pathol 36:29–33

4. Maurel S, Toquin D, Briand FX et al (2011) First full-length sequences of the S gene of European isolates reveal further diversity among turkey coronaviruses. Avian Pathol 40:179–189

5. Chen YN, Wu CC, Lin TL (2011) Identification and characterization of a neutralizing-epitope-containing spike protein fragment in turkey coronavirus. Arch Virol 156:1525–1535

6. Howard MW, Travanty EA, Jeffers SA et al (2008) Aromatic amino acids in the juxtamembrane domain of severe acute respiratory syndrome coronavirus spike glycoprotein are important for receptor dependent virus entry and cell–cell fusion. J Virol 82:2883–2894

7. Loa CC, Lin TL, Wu CC et al (2006) Differential detection of turkey coronavirus, infectious bronchitis virus, and bovine coronavirus by a multiplex polymerase chain reaction. J Virol Methods 131:86–91

8. Breslin JJ, Smith LG, Barnes HJ et al (2000) Comparison of virus isolation, immunohistochemistry, and reverse transcriptase polymerase chain reaction procedures for detection of turkey coronavirus. Avian Dis 44:624–631

9. Holland PM, Abramson RD, Watson R et al (1991) Detection of specific polymerase chain reaction product by utilizing the 50–30 exonuclease activity of *Thermus aquaticus* DNA polymerase. Proc Natl Acad Sci U S A 88:7276–7280

10. Chen Y-N, Wu CC, Bryan T et al (2010) Specific real time reverse transcription polymerase chain reaction for detection and quantitation of turkey coronavirus RNA in tissues and feces from turkeys infected with turkey coronavirus. J Virol Methods 163:452–458

Chapter 14

PCR Amplification and Sequencing Analysis of Full-Length Turkey Coronavirus Spike Gene

Yi-Ning Chen, Aydemir Akin, Chien Chang Loa, Mustafa Ababneh, Jianzhong Cao, Wan-Jung Chen, Ching Ching Wu, and Tsang Long Lin

Abstract

Turkey coronaviral enteritis caused by turkey coronavirus (TCoV) continues to infect turkey flocks, resulting in significant economic loss. Determining and understanding genetic relationships among different TCoV isolates or strains is important for controlling the disease. Using two-step RT-PCR assays that amplify the full length of TCoV spike (S) gene, TCoV isolates can be sequenced, analyzed, and genotyped. Described in this chapter is the protocol on PCR amplification and sequencing analysis of full-length TCoV S gene. Such protocol is useful in molecular epidemiology for establishing an effective strategy to control the transmission of TCoV among turkey flocks.

Key words Turkey coronavirus, Spike gene, Sequencing, Genotype

1 Introduction

Turkey coronaviral enteritis caused by turkey coronavirus (TCoV) has been reported with varied severity in clinical signs in the affected turkey flocks from different states in the USA [1, 2], Canada [3], Brazil [4], and Europe [5]. The major clinical signs of TCoV infection include depression, ruffled feathers, watery diarrhea, decreased body weight gain, and uneven flock growth. The most striking gross lesions are markedly distended intestine with gaseous and watery content, especially in the ileum and ceca. The salient histopathologic findings include shortening of the intestinal villi, increase in crypt depth, and widening of intervillous spaces [1]. TCoV belongs to species *Avian coronavirus* of the genus *Gammacoronavirus* in the family *Coronaviridae*. The genome of TCoV is a linear positive-sense single-stranded RNA encoding three major structural proteins, including spike (S), membrane (M), and nucleocapsid (N) protein. While M and N genes are conserved, S gene is a more common target used for

Leyi Wang (ed.), *Animal Coronaviruses*, Springer Protocols Handbooks,
DOI 10.1007/978-1-4939-3414-0_14, © Springer Science+Business Media New York 2016

coronavirus (CoV) differentiation because S gene is highly variable among different CoVs. The S gene sequences among different TCoV isolates (93–99.7 %) are relatively conserved as compared to different infectious bronchitis virus (IBV) strains, although both TCoV and IBV belong to the same species *Avian coronavirus* [6–8]. Because the pair-wise comparison of S gene sequences revealed only 34 % of similarity between TCoV isolates and IBV strains while the remaining 3′-end encoding region shared over 80 % of similarity, it has been suggested that TCoV arose through a recombination of S gene from IBV [6, 9–11].

A protocol for PCR amplification, sequencing, and sequence analysis of TCoV S gene for genotyping of TCoV isolates based on TCoV S gene sequences is highlighted in this chapter. In **step 1**, intestine tissues are collected from TCoV-infected turkeys and TCoV is purified through ultracentrifugation on continuous sucrose gradient. In **step 2**, TCoV RNA is extracted from intestines and reverse transcribed to cDNA. In **step 3**, the full-length S gene of TCoV is amplified and sequenced. In **step 4**, the nucleotide sequence of the full-length S gene of TCoV is assembled from 12 sequence fragments flanking the entire length of S gene. The S gene sequences of TCoV isolates and those from other coronaviruses published in GenBank are further analyzed by alignment and phylogenetic tree and thus TCoV genotypes are determined.

2   Materials

2.1   Turkey Coronavirus Preparation

2.1.1   Reagent

1. Antiserum against TCoV/IN540/94 (GenBank accession number EU022525).

2. Phosphate-buffered saline (PBS) is composed of 1.44 g Na_2HPO_4, 8 g NaCl, 0.24 g KH_2PO_4, and 0.2 g KCl in 1 L ddH_2O. The solution is adjusted to pH 7.2 and autoclaved before use.

3. Whatman 0.45 and 0.22 μm syringe filter (Thermo Fisher Scientific, Waltham, MA, USA).

4. Thin-wall polypropylene ultracentrifuge tubes, open-top, transparent, 17 mL with 16×102 mm for rotor SW28 of Optima XL-100 K ultracentrifuge (Beckman Coulter, Fullerton, CA, USA).

5. RNApure™ reagent (GenHunter, Nashville, TN, USA).

6. Diethyl pyrocarbonate (DEPC) (Sigma-Aldrich, St. Louis, MO, USA): DEPC is very sensitive to moisture, so it needs to be stored at 2–8 °C to help reduce exposure to moisture.

7. Preparation of DEPC-treated water (DEPC-H_2O):

   (a) Prepare 0.1 % (v/v) DEPC in the water undergone reverse osmosis filtration and deionization. Add 0.1 mL DEPC solution to 100 mL of water. DEPC appears as globules and needs continuous stirring until the globules disappear. It takes 12 h at 37 °C in a fume hood. DEPC can dissolve plastic, so it is better to store DEPC solution in a glass bottle.

(b) Autoclave 0.1 % DEPC solution at 121 °C for 15 min to remove any trace of DEPC. The autoclaved DEPC-H_2O can be stored at any temperature.

2.1.2 Equipment

1. Bio-Gen Pro200 homogenizer (Pro Scientific, Oxford, CT, USA).

2. Optima XL-100K ultracentrifuge (Beckman Coulter, Fullerton, CA, USA).

3. Bio-Rad Model 395 Gradient former (Bio-Rad, Hercules, CA, USA).

4. GeneQuant 1300 Spectrophotometer (GE Healthcare Bio-Sciences, Piscataway, NJ, USA).

2.2 RNA Extraction and cDNA Preparation

2.2.1 Reagent

1. SuperScript® III reverse transcriptase (Invitrogen™, Life Technologies, Grand Island, NY, USA).

2.3 PCR Amplification and Sequencing

2.3.1 Reagent

1. *Taq* DNA polymerase (Promega, Madison, WI, USA).

2. *Pfu* DNA polymerase (Stratagene™, Agilent Technologies, La Jolla, CA, USA).

3. Primers can be synthesized by Integrated DNA Technologies (IDT, San Jose, CA, USA) or other equivalent companies. The primers and sequence information are listed in Table 1. The lyophilized powders of products prepared by company are to be dissolved in DEPC-H_2O to 100 μM as stock solution (100×). The working solution of primers is 10 μM. Both stock and working solution of primers are stored at −20 °C.

4. Zymoclean™ gel DNA recovery kit (Zymo, Irvine, CA, USA).

5. TOPO® TA Cloning® Kit with pCR®II-TOPO® Vector and One Shot® TOP10F′ Chemically Competent E. coli (Invitrogen™, Life Technologies, Grand Island, NY, USA).

6. DNAstar Lasergene® software (DNASTAR, Madison, WI, USA).

2.3.2 Equipment

1. Applied Biosystems® GeneAmp® PCR System Thermal Cyclers (Life Technologies, Grand Island, NY, USA).

Table 1
Oligonucleotide primers and sequences used for turkey coronavirus spike gene polymerase chain reaction and sequencing

	Name	5′ → 3′ sequence	Position[a]	Orient
PCR primers	Sup	TGAAAACTGAACAAAAGACAGACT	−63 to −4	+
	Sdown3	TTTGTTGAATTATTTGCTGACCA	3813–3835	−
Sequencing primers	AS-cor	CCAAACATACCAAGGCCACTT	3392–3413	+
	S101F1	TAATTTAACATGGGGCAACT	410–429	+
	S101F2	TTCCCTAAAGTTAAAAGTGTT	459–479	−
	S101R1	CTGTCTAAATATGATGCCACTTCC	2985–3008	−
	S101R2	GGGCATTACACCATACTTTCCAGA	2955–2978	+
	S102F1	AAGTTGTGTATATTAGGGCTGAA	936–959	+
	S102F2	TTTATACGCAACATTCAT	982–999	−
	S102R1	TTACACTCTCAAAACCTCTA	2501–2520	−
	S102R2	ACCTCTAGCTACTTCAACAAATCC	2484–2507	+
	S103F1	ACCGTGCCAGACAGTTTCA	1439–1457	+
	S103F2	GAGTTTTGTAGGCTTGTTTCTTC	1481–1503	−
	S103R1	GTAGAACAAGCGACAAATCAAACC	2035–2058	−

[a]The positions of primers were relative to the start codon of nucleotide sequence of TCoV/IN/540/94 (EU022525)

3   Methods

3.1   Turkey Coronavirus Preparation

3.1.1   Clinical Sample Collection and Virus Propagation

1. Field cases of turkey coronaviral enteritis are diagnosed by clinical signs, gross lesions, histopathologic findings, immunofluorescence antibody (IFA) assay with antiserum against TCoV/IN540/94, electron microscopy, and reverse transcription polymerase chain reaction (RT-PCR) targeting partial fragment of N or S gene.

2. Homogenize the intestines from TCoV-infected turkeys with 5 volumes of chill sterile PBS on ice using Bio-Gen Pro200 homogenizer (*see* **Note 1**).

3. Centrifuge the homogenate at $1449 \times g$ for 10 min at 4 °C.

4. Filter the supernatant without any tissue debris through Whatman 0.45 and 0.22 μm syringe filters, respectively.

5. Inoculate the filtrate into the amniotic cavity of 22-day-old embryonated turkey eggs.

6. Harvest turkey embryo intestines after 3 days of incubation at 99.3 °F with humidity of 56 %.

7. Repeat the procedures of virus propagation in 22-day-old embryonated turkey eggs up to five times serially, if needed.

3.1.2 Turkey Coronavirus Purification

1. Homogenate three harvested turkey embryonic intestines after TCoV propagation described in Sect. 3.1.1 with 15 mL of chill sterile PBS on ice using Bio-Gen Pro200 homogenizer.

2. Centrifuge the homogenate at 3000 rpm for 10 min at 4 °C.

3. Layer about 10 mL of the supernatant on top of 4 mL of 30 % sucrose (middle layer) and followed by 2 mL of 60 % sucrose (bottom layer) in a 17 mL ultracentrifuge tube for rotor SW28. The total volume needs to be about 80–90 % height of the ultracentrifuge tube or the tube may crush after ultracentrifugation.

4. Centrifuge the sample by ultracentrifugation in rotor SW28 at $103,679 \times g$ for 3 h at 4 °C in Optima XL-100K ultracentrifuge.

5. Collect the interface between 30 % sucrose and 60 % sucrose with 10 mL pipet gently and carefully. Add PBS to the collected interface materials till the maximum volume of 5 mL and suspend the materials containing TCoV thoroughly.

6. Place 5 mL of interface materials on top of 10 mL of continuous 40–60 % sucrose gradient (*see* **Note 2**).

7. Centrifuge the sample with sucrose gradient by ultracentrifugation in rotor SW28 at 24,000 rpm at 4 °C for 20 h.

8. Collect the TCoV-containing band of buoyant density 1.16–1.24 g/mL as the viral stock and save it in the −80 °C freezer or liquid nitrogen until used.

3.2 RNA Extraction and cDNA Preparation

3.2.1 Total RNA Extraction

1. Take 200 µL of purified TCoV and mix with 1 mL of RNApure™ reagent in a 1.7 mL microcentrifuge tube.

2. Vortex briefly to dissolve any debris completely. Incubate at 4 °C for 10 min.

3. Add 180 µL of chloroform. Vortex the tube for 10 s. Incubate the tube at 4 °C for 10 min. Centrifuge the tube at $13,000 \times g$ at 4 °C for 10 min.

4. Take the upper colorless aqueous phase to a new 1.7 mL microcentrifuge tube.

5. Add equal volume (about 0.5 mL) of cold isopropyl alcohol and vortex the tube for 10 s. Incubate the tube at 4 °C for 10 min.

6. Centrifuge the tube at $13,000 \times g$ at 4 °C for 10 min. Discard the supernatant.

7. Wash the RNA pellet with 1 mL of 70 % ethanol by resuspending the pellet and centrifuge at $13,000 \times g$ at 4 °C for 2 min. Discard the supernatant.

8. Air-dry the RNA pellet with the tube upside down for 1 min.

9. Dissolve the RNA pellet with 30 µL of DEPC-H_2O and measure the concentration of RNA using GeneQuant 1300 Spectrophotometer.

3.2.2 Reverse Transcription

1. Obtain cDNA from the extracted RNA by reverse transcription (RT) using SuperScript® III reverse transcriptase. In the first reaction, add 1 μL of random hexamer primer (50–100 ng/μL) into 9 μL of RNA (9–15 μg), incubate at 70 °C for 3 min, and quickly chill in ice. Briefly centrifuge the tube and proceed the second reaction. Add 4 μL of 5× reaction buffer, 2 μL of DTT (0.1 M), 2 μL of dNTPs (10 mM each dATP, dTTP, dCTP, dGTP), 1 μL of RNaseOUT™ (40 U), and 1 μL of SuperScript™ III reverse transcriptase (200 U) into the first reaction solution. Incubate the second reaction at room temperature for 5 min and 50 °C for 1 h and inactivate at 70 °C for 15 min.

3.3 PCR Amplification and Sequencing

1. Amplify the full-length TCoV S gene (about 3.9 kb) by PCR with the primers Sup and Sdown3 (Table 1) and the mixture of *Taq* DNA polymerase and *Pfu* DNA polymerase in a ratio of volume:volume = 64:1.

2. Prepare 50 μL of PCR reaction mixture (Table 2).

3. Perform PCR reaction in an Applied Biosystems® GeneAmp® PCR System Thermal Cycler 9700 according to the cycling program: 94 °C for 5 min and 40 cycles of 94 °C for 1 min, 55 °C for 4 min, and 72 °C for 10 min, and then stop at 4 °C for storage.

4. Electrophorese the PCR product on 1 % agarose gel to confirm the size (about 3.9 kb) and purity of the PCR product amplified by the primers Sup and Sdown3.

5. Purify Sup/Sdown3 PCR product from agarose gel by Zymoclean™ gel DNA recovery kit for sequencing.

Table 2
Reaction mixture for polymerase chain reaction amplifying the full length of turkey coronavirus spike gene

Components	Volume (μL)
cDNA	1
10× Reaction mix	5
dNTPs (10 mM each)	1
MgCl₂ (25 mM)	3
Taq:*Pfu* DNA polymerase (v:v = 64:1)	1
Forward primer Sup 10 μM	1
Reverse primer Sdown 10 μM	1
DEPC H₂O	37
Total volume	50

6. Obtain the nucleotide sequences of the purified Sup/Sdown3 PCR product by sequencing using the 12 sequencing primers listed in Table 1 at a certified genomics facility.

7. Clone the purified Sup/Sdown3 PCR product into pCR®II-TOPO® plasmid vector and transform it into *Escherichia coli* strain One Shot® TOP10F′ for storage purpose (*see* **Note 3**).

3.4 Sequence Analysis

1. Assemble 12 nucleotide sequences from 12 sequencing primers (Table 1) to obtain the full length of TCoV S gene by using DNAstar Lasergene® software.

2. Analyze the full-length S genes from different TCoV field isolates by Clustal W alignment method using DNAstar Lasergene® software or Web-based MEGA6 program (http://www.megasoftware.net). Sequence alignment can arrange the sequences of DNA and deduced amino acids to identify regions of similarity resulting from evolutionary relationships among the compared sequences.

(a) Open MEGA6 program, click "Align" on the tool bar, choose "Edit/Build Alignment," check the option of "create a new alignment" in the first dialog box, push "OK," and then choose either "DNA" or "Protein" sequence alignment, and the Alignment Explorer window will open.

(b) There are three ways to add sequences into alignment program. For the first two ways, go to "Edit" menu and click either "Insert Blank Sequence" to key in each sequence manually or "Insert Sequence From File" to import the selected sequences in Text (*.txt, *.seq) or FASTA file formats. For the third way, go to "Web" menu and click "Query GenBank" to import Web-based sequences by checking the "Add to Alignment" option for each interested sequence.

(c) After all sequences for alignment are added, go to "Edit" menu in the Alignment Explorer window to select all sequences for alignment, and then go to "Alignment" menu to select "Align by Clustal W (Codons)" for the process of alignment. Choose Align Codons for DNA alignment to avoid introducing gaps into positions that would result in frame shifts in the real sequences. Use the default settings of Clustal W method for DNA alignment but change the Multiple Alignment Gap Opening penalty to 3 and the Multiple Alignment Gap Extension penalty to 1.8 for protein alignment. When the alignment is complete, go to "Data" menu and choose "Save Session" to save the alignment result as Aln session (*.mas) format. For further construct of phylogenetic tree, go to "Data":

menu and click "Export Alignment" to choose "MEGA Format" to save the alignment result as .meg extension.

3. A phylogenetic tree can be constructed by many methods used widely and maximum likelihood (ML) method is chosen based on previous coronaviral studies.

(a) ML uses a variety of substitution models to correct for multiple changes at the same site during the evolutionary history of the sequences, like Tamura 3-parameter and Kimura 2-parameter models, and the best model to use for each analysis can be calculated by MEGA6 program. Go to MEGA6 main window and choose "Models" to select "Find Best DNA/Protein Models (ML)." Choose the alignment file saved before for calculation. Note the preferred model to construct a phylogenetic tree based on the list of models in order of preferences.

(b) Go to MEGA6 main window and choose "Phylogeny" to select "Construct/Test Maximum Likelihood Tree." Fill in the parameters of "Model/Method" and "Rates among Sites" based on the preferred parameters calculated previously in the preference dialog appearing. Select "Partial Deletion" in "Gap/Missing Data Treatment" to avoid losing too much information. Set "No. of Bootstrap Replicates" to 1000 under "Phylogeny Test" to estimate the reliability of the tree.

(c) After computing, a tree explorer window will open the tree. Save the tree as a (*.mts) file, choose "Export Current Tree (Newick)" from "File" menu for further modification in other tree drawing program, choose "Save as PDF File" from "Image" menu for graphic file format accepted for publishing, or choose "Save as PNG File" or "Save as Enhanced Meta File" for further process.

4   Notes

1. Put the turkey intestines containing TCoV in 50 mL tube. If the volume of intestines reaches 5 mL mark of 50 mL tube, add 25 mL (5 volumes) of chill sterile PBS for homogenization. It is recommended to homogenize the intestine tissue for 30 s and cool the tube in ice in cycles until the intestine tissue is homogenized thoroughly because the heat produced by the process of homogenization can damage the integrity of RNA in intestine tissues.

2. To prepare 40–60 % sucrose continuous gradient, Bio-Rad Model 395 Gradient former or equivalent gradient maker is used. Put 5 mL of 40 % sucrose and 5 mL of 60 % sucrose in

two connected compartments of Gradient former, respectively. Place a stirrer bar in the compartment with 40 % sucrose (lower extreme concentration of sucrose gradient). There is a valve to control the connection between two compartments and a plastic tube leading to an ultracentrifuge tube (Beckman Coulter) from the compartment with 40 % sucrose. Put the Gradient former on top of magnetic stirrer. Open the stirrer and wait till the stirrer bar stir steady and then open the valve. Collect the mixed sucrose in an ultracentrifuge tube to get 10 mL of 40–60 % sucrose continuous gradient.

3. To increase the successful rate of TA cloning, a 3′ A-overhangs post-amplification is performed. Add *Taq* polymerase buffer, dATP (10 mM), and 0.5 U of *Taq* polymerase to the purified PCR product. Incubate the reaction for 10–15 min at 72 °C. For further TA cloning, mix 1 μL of pCRII-TOPO vector, 1 μL of Salt Solution provided by the kit, and 4 μL of the purified PCR product gently and incubate the reaction at room temperature for 30 min. For further transformation, add 2 μL of TA cloning reaction to 50 μL of Top10F′ *E. coli* and incubate on ice for 30 min. Heat-shock the cells for 30 s at 42 °C without shaking and transfer the cells to ice immediately. Add 250 μL of room temperature S.O.C. medium provided by the kit. Cap the tube tightly and shake the tube horizontally (200 rpm) at 37 °C for 1 h. Spread 10–50 μL from the transformation on a pre-warmed selective plate and incubate overnight at 37 °C. To ensure even spreading of small volumes, add 20 μL of super optimal broth with catabolite repression (S.O.C.) medium (Sigma-Aldrich). Pick about ten white or light blue colonies for analysis. Do not pick dark blue colonies.

Acknowledgement

The protocol "PCR amplification and sequencing analysis of full-length turkey coronavirus spike gene" outlined in this chapter had been successfully carried out in the authors' studies on molecular diagnostics, molecular virology, immunology, and/or vaccinology of turkey coronavirus infection. Those studies were in part financially supported by USDA, North Carolina Poultry Federation, and/or Indiana Department of Agriculture and technically assisted by Drs. Tom Bryan and David Hermes, Mr. Tom Hooper, and Ms. Donna Schrader for clinical investigation, virus isolation and propagation, and animal experimentation.

References

1. Lin TL, Loa CC, Tsai SC et al (2002) Characterization of turkey coronavirus from turkey poults with acute enteritis. Vet Microbiol 84:179–186

2. Day JM, Gonder E, Jennings S et al (2014) Investigating turkey enteric coronavirus circulating in the Southeastern United States and Arkansas during 2012 and 2013. Avian Dis 58:313–317

3. Gomaa MH, Yoo D, Ojkic D et al (2009) Infection with a pathogenic turkey coronavirus isolate negatively affects growth performance and intestinal morphology of young turkey poults in Canada. Avian Pathol 38:279–286

4. Teixeira MC, Luvizotto MC, Ferrari HF et al (2007) Detection of turkey coronavirus in commercial turkey poults in Brazil. Avian Pathol 36:29–33

5. Maurel S, Toquin D, Briand FX et al (2011) First full-length sequences of the S gene of European isolates reveal further diversity among turkey coronaviruses. Avian Pathol 40:179–189

6. Loa CC, Wu CC, Lin TL (2006) Comparison of 3′-end encoding regions of turkey coronavirus isolates from Indiana, North Carolina, and Minnesota with chicken infectious bronchitis coronavirus strains. Intervirology 49:230–238

7. Wang CH, Huang YC (2000) Relationship between serotypes and genotypes based on the hypervariable region of the S1 gene of infectious bronchitis virus. Arch Virol 145:291–300

8. Lin TL, Loa CC, Wu CC et al (2002) Antigenic relationship of turkey coronavirus isolates from different geographic locations in the United States. Avian Dis 46:466–472

9. Cao J, Wu CC, Lin TL (2008) Complete nucleotide sequence of polyprotein gene 1 and genome organization of turkey coronavirus. Virus Res 136(1–2):43–49

10. Jackwood MW, Boynton TO, Hilt DA et al (2009) Emergence of a group 3 coronavirus through recombination. Virology 398:98–108

11. Hughes AL (2011) Recombinational histories of avian infectious bronchitis virus and turkey coronavirus. Arch Virol 156:1823–1829

Chapter 15

Feline Coronavirus RT-PCR Assays for Feline Infectious Peritonitis Diagnosis

Takehisa Soma

Abstract

Feline infectious peritonitis (FIP) is a highly fatal systemic disease in cats, caused by feline coronavirus (FCoV) infection. FCoV usually has little clinical significance; however, a mutation of this avirulent virus (feline enteric coronavirus) to a virulent type (FIP virus) can lead to FIP incidence. It is difficult to diagnose FIP, since the viruses cannot be distinguished using serological or virological methods. Recently, genetic techniques, such as RT-PCR, have been conducted for FIP diagnosis. In this chapter, the reliability of RT-PCR and procedures used to determine FCoV infection as part of antemortem FIP diagnosis is described.

Key words Diagnosis, Feline coronavirus, Feline infectious peritonitis, RT-PCR

1 Introduction

Feline infectious peritonitis (FIP) is an immune-mediated progressive and systemic infectious disease occurring in domestic cats and wild felids, and caused by infection with feline coronavirus (FCoV), a single-stranded RNA virus, which has been classified as *Alphacoronavirus* along with canine coronavirus (CCoV) and transmissible gastroenteritis virus [1, 2]. FCoV is transmitted by the fecal-oral route and usually causes a mild to inapparent enteritis [2]. FIP is considered to be induced by a virulent mutant (FIP virus; FIPV) of this enteric FCoV (feline enteric coronavirus; FECV) [2, 3]. The incidence of FIP is generally as low as 1–3 % in FCoV-infected cats, though it varies depending on age, breed, environment, and superinfection with other viruses [2, 4–6].

It is divided into two basic clinical forms, effusive FIP, in which effusion is observed in the body cavity, and non-effusive FIP, in which multiple pyogranuloma lesions are observed, though differences in lesions are influenced by individual immunity [7]. Furthermore, there are two types (I and II) of FCoV, with FCoV type II considered to arise by a recombination of FCoV type I and

Leyi Wang (ed.), *Animal Coronaviruses*, Springer Protocols Handbooks,
DOI 10.1007/978-1-4939-3414-0_15, © Springer Science+Business Media New York 2016

CCoV [8–10]. Based on genetic and serological investigations, FCoV type I is overwhelmingly dominant as compared to type II and mixed infection with both types is not rare [11–14].

Since FIPV and FECV cannot be fully distinguished using serological methods, it is generally difficult to diagnose FIP [1]. Therefore, other laboratory findings such as hematology and serum biochemistry examinations [15, 16] have been referred to FIP diagnosis. Recently, it has been stated that demonstration of FCoV RNA by RT-PCR is one of the most reliable diagnostic indicators of FIP in suspected cases [7, 17]. However, FIPV and FECV are not necessarily distinguished with certainty, and the reliability of RT-PCR for FIP diagnosis depends largely on the test specimens as well as rearing environment of the affected cat.

Test specimens used with FCoV RT-PCR for FIP diagnosis include body cavity fluid (ascitic and pleural effusions), blood, cerebrospinal fluid (CSF), and tissues. As shown in Table 1, effusion is the most suitable, and FCoV RNA detection provides highly sensitive and specific diagnosis [1, 17–19]. When using CSF, RNA detection can also give a highly specific diagnosis. However, the absence of FIP cannot be generally concluded based on negative results, because small amounts of the virus may exist in CSF from FIP cases [1, 20, 21]. Even in non-FIP and healthy carriers, RNA may be detected in blood for several months after FECV infection [22, 23]. Of note, associated RNA is frequently detected in blood from FCoV-endemic multi-cat households. Thus, the reliability of RT-PCR-positive results obtained from a blood specimen is dependent on the rearing environment [23–25]. In contrast, FIP may be excluded when a blood specimen is RT-PCR negative, because the RNA detection sensitivity is relatively high with blood from FIP cases [17, 23, 26, 27]. RNA detection sensitivity varies among tissues, i.e., higher in the liver and spleen, and lower in the kidneys and heart [28–30]. Tissue samples generally contain blood, which compromises the reproducibility of FIP diagnosis with RT-PCR-positive tissues [1, 29].

In this chapter, three RT-PCR techniques generally employed for FIP diagnosis in Japan are outlined in regard to their usefulness for antemortem diagnosis.

Table 1
Predictive values of FCoV RT-PCR in FIP diagnosis

Predictive value	Effusion	Blood	CSF	Tissue
Positive (specificity)	High	Valuable	High	Valuable
Negative (sensitivity)	High	Moderate to high	Low	Valuable

2   Materials

2.1   Primer Set for RT-PCR

Three FCoV RT-PCR primer sets are recommended for FIP diagnosis, as shown in Table 2. One targets the 3′-untranslated region (3′-UTR) (P205–P211 primer set) [17] for FIP screening. This region is the first choice for RT-PCR, because it is highly conserved among *Alphacoronavirus* and allows sensitive FCoV RNA detection. A second-round (nested) PCR primer set (P276–P204) is also available to check the specificity of the RT-PCR result.

To confirm a positive RT-PCR reaction, a subsequent RT-PCR assay is recommended using a primer set that recognizes subgenomic mRNA of the M gene (212–1179 primer set) [27] (Table 2). Since detection of this gene indicates viral replication, FIPV, which has increased microphage infectivity, is able to be detected with high specificity. This RT-PCR technique is more useful for specimens other than effusion samples and CSF. However, in our experience, mRNA detection tends to be less sensitive than 3′-UTR RT-PCR.

To determine the type of cases shown positive with the above RT-PCR assays, a primer set targeting the S gene should be used for a multiplex RT-PCR (Iffs-Icfs-Iubs primer set) (Table 2) [31]. For negative cases shown by RT-PCR, nested PCR should be conducted using nIffle-nIcfs-nIubs primer set (*see* **Note 1**).

Table 2
Primers for the amplification of FCoV gene

Primer	Sequence (5′–3′)	Orientation	Target	Product size	Reference
P205	GGCAACCCGATGTTTAAAACTGG	Sense	3′-UTR	223 bp	[17]
P211	CACTAGATCCAGACGTTAGCTC	Antisense			
P276	CCGAGGAATTACTGGTCATCGCG	Sense		177 bp	
P204	GCTCTTCCATTGTTGGCTCGTC	Antisense			
212	TAATGCCATACACGAACCAGCT	Sense	M (mRNA)	295 bp	[27]
1179	GTGCTAGATTTGTCTTCGGACACC	Antisense			
Iffs	GTTTCAACCTAGAAAGCCTCAGAT	Sense	S	Type I 376 bp	[31]
Icfs	GCCTAGTATTATACCTGACTA	Sense		Type II 283 bp	
Iubs	CCACACATACCAAGGCC	Antisense			
nIffles	CCTAGAAAGCCTCAGATGAGTG	Sense		Type I 360 bp	
nIcfs	CAGACCAAACTGGACTGTAC	Sense		Type II 218 bp	
nIubs	CCAAGGCCATTTTACATA	Antisense			

Representative positive reaction bands from these three RT-PCR methods and two nested PCR assays are as shown in Figs. 1 and 2.

2.2 Reagent for FCoV RT-PCR

2.2.1 Extraction and Purification of Viral RNA

1. QIAamp Viral RNA Mini Kit (Qiagen).
2. QIAamp Blood RNA Mini Kit (Qiagen).
3. RNeasy Mini Kit (Qiagen).
4. DNase- and RNase-free water (Invitrogen).
5. DNase- and RNase-free ethanol, 99.5 %(V/V) (Wako).

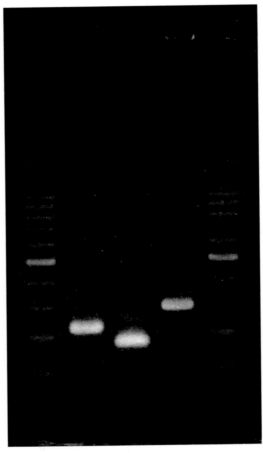

Fig. 1 Agarose gel electrophoresis of products obtained by FCoV RT-PCR targeting 3′-UTR and M (mRNA) genes. Lane 1: 3′-UTR RT-PCR (first-round PCR) (223 bp), lane 2: 3′-UTR nested PCR (177 bp), lane 3: M (mRNA) RT-PCR (295 bp), L: 100 bp DNA ladder marker

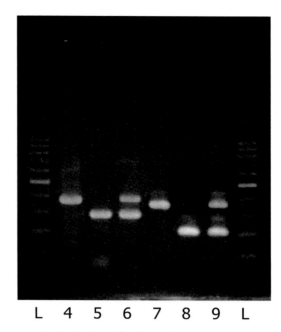

Fig. 2 Agarose gel electrophoresis of products obtained by FCoV multiplex RT-PCR targeting S gene. Lanes 4–6: RT-PCR (first-round PCR), Lanes 7–9: nested PCR, Lanes 4 and 7: Type I (376 bp and 360 bp, respectively), Lanes 5 and 8: Type II (283 bp and 218 bp, respectively), Lanes 6 and 9: Both type infections,, L: 100 bp DNA ladder marker

2.2.2 RT-PCR	1. Qiagen One-Step RT-PCR kit, containing 5× RT-PCR buffer, enzyme mix, and dNTP mix (10 mM each) (Qiagen).
	2. RNase inhibitor, 40 U/mL (Promega).
	3. Primers, 10 μM (shown in Table 2).
2.2.3 Second-Round (Nested) PCR	1. DNase- and RNase-free water (invitrogen).
	2. AmpliTaq Gold DNA polymerase, 5 U/mL, with 10× PCR buffer, MgCl₂ solution (25 mM), and dNTP mix (2 mM each) (Applied Biosystems).
	3. Primers, 10 μM (shown in Table 2).
2.2.4 Agarose Gel Electrophoresis	1. Tris-borate-EDTA (TBE) buffer, pH 8.3 (TaKaRa).
	2. Agarose-LE powder (Ambion).
	3. 6× Gel loading dye, containing bromophenol blue and orange G (Toyobo).
	4. 100 bp DNA ladder marker, with loading dye (Toyobo).
2.2.5 EtBr Staining	1. Ethidium bromide (EtBr), 10 mg/mL (invitrogen).
	2. Distilled water (for diluting EtBr stock solution), not necessarily DNase- and RNase-free water.

3   Methods

3.1   RNA Extraction and Purification

Viral RNA is extracted from effusion, serum, plasma, whole blood, cerebrospinal fluid (CSF), and tissue (biopsy) specimens using a QIAamp Viral RNA Mini Kit, QIAamp Blood RNA Mini Kit, or RNeasy Mini Kit (Qiagen), according to the manufacturer's instructions (*see* **Notes 2–6**).

3.2   RT-PCR

Next, reaction mixtures for RT-PCR are prepared, as shown in Table 3. Five microliters of the template (purified RNA) is added to the reaction mixture and subjected to amplification in a thermal cycler (Table 4) (*see* **Notes 7–9**).

Table 3
Reaction mixtures for FCoV RT-PCR

	Primer set	
Component	**P205–P211, 212–1179**	**Iffs-Icfs-Iubs**
DNase-free, RNase-free water	27.8 μL	26.3 μL
5× QIAGEN OneStep RT-PCR Buffer	10.0 μL	10.0 μL
dNTP mix (containing 10 mM of each dNTP)	2.0 μL	2.0 μL
10 μM Primers	1.5 μL each	1.5 μL each
QIAGEN OneStep RT-PCR enzyme mix	2.0 μL	2.0 μL
RNase inhibitor (10 U/μL)	0.2 μL	0.2 μL
Total volume	45.0 μL	45.0 μL

Table 4
Reaction conditions for FCoV RT-PCR

	Primer set		
	P205-P211	**212–1179**	**Iffs-Icfs-Iubs**
Reverse transcription	50 °C for 30 min	50 °C for 30 min	50 °C for 30 min
Inactivation of reverse transcriptase and denaturation of cDNA template	95 °C for 15 min	95 °C for 15 min	95 °C for 15 min
(Sequential cycle)	(40 cycles)	(30 cycles)	(35 cycles)
Denaturation	94 °C for 50 s	94 °C for 1 min	94 °C for 1 min
Annealing	55 °C for 1 min	62 °C for 1 min	50 °C for 1 min
Extension	72 °C for 1 min	72 °C for 1 min	72 °C for 1 min
Final extension	72 °C for 7 min	72 °C for 7 min	72 °C for 7 min

3.3 Second-Round (Nested) PCR

Reaction mixtures for the nested PCR assay are then prepared, as shown in Table 5. Five microliters of the RT-PCR product diluted 100 times with DNase- and RNase-free water is added to the reaction mixtures, and then subjected to amplification (Table 6) (*see* **Notes 7–9**).

3.4 Agarose Gel Electrophoresis

Five microliters of the PCR product is then added to 6× gel loading dye at a 1/6 volume ratio and electrophoresed with TBE buffer at 100 V for 35 min on a 2 % agarose gel at room temperature.

3.5 EtBr Staining

Following electrophoresis, the gel is immersed into 10 mg/mL of EtBr solution. After staining for 30–40 min, the gel is photographed under UV illumination (*see* **Notes 10–12**).

Table 5
Reaction mixtures for FCoV nested PCR

	Primer set	
Component	P276–P204	nIffles-nIcfs-nIubs
DNase- and RNase-free water	29.8 μL	27.75 μL
10× PCR buffer (containing no MgCl₂)	5.0 μL	5.0 μL
25 mM MgCl₂	3.0 μL	4.0 μL
dNTP mix (containing 2 mM of each dNTP)	5.0 μL	5.0 μL
10 μM Primers	1.0 μL each	1.0 μL each
Taq polymerase (5 U/μL)	0.2 μL	0.25 μL
Total volume	45.0 μL	45.0 μL

Table 6
Reaction conditions for FCoV nested PCR

	Primer set	
	P276–P204	nIffles-nIcfs-nIubs
Initial denaturation		90 °C for 5 min
(Sequential cycle)	(35 cycles)	(35 cycles)
Denaturation	94 °C for 50 sec	94 °C for 1 min
Annealing	55 °C for 1 min	47 °C for 1 min
Extension	72 °C for 1 min	72 °C for 1 min
Final extension	72 °C for 7 min	72 °C for 7 min

4   Notes

For FCoV RT-PCR implementation and FIP diagnosis, the following points should be noted.

1. False-negative results may be obtained when no viral RNA is detected with the indicated primers because of viral mutations. This is more likely to occur with primers targeting the S gene.

2. Care should be exercised to prevent coagulation of whole blood samples. EDTA is suitable as an anticoagulant, while heparin is not recommended, because it may cause coagulation during transportation.

3. Care should be exercised to prevent blood contamination during CSF sampling, as viral RNA may be contained in blood even in non-FIP cases.

4. Care should be exercised during sampling and transportation, because RNA is fragile, and disposable DNase- and RNase-free sampling containers should be used. Collected samples should be immediately transported to a laboratory in a refrigerated state.

5. DNase- and RNase-free phosphate buffer saline (PBS) should be used to increase sample volume before testing as needed.

6. Effusion, serum, and plasma specimens should be centrifuged with a refrigerated centrifuge prior to purification with the QIAamp Viral RNA Mini Kit, and the resulting supernatants should then be purified.

7. Reaction mixtures should be prepared and dispensed on ice.

8. PCR is highly sensitive and may yield false-positive results when contaminated by even a small amount of nucleic acid. Thus, reaction mixtures should be prepared and dispensed in clean environments, such as a clean bench, and only test results obtained by skilled experimenters are considered to be reliable.

9. Only DNase- and RNase-free instruments, such as test tubes and pipette chips, should be used.

10. Since EtBr is deactivated by light, its solution should be stored in a light-shielded condition.

11. Care should be exercised in handling EtBr for gel staining, because EtBr is toxic to humans. It should be also detoxified in appropriate manners, such as activated carbon adsorption, reductive decomposition, and oxidative decomposition, before disposal. A detoxifying reagent is commercially available (EtBr destroyer, Wako).

12. Care should be exercised in regard to UV irradiation during gel observation, as UV may damage eyes and skin.

References

1. Addie DD (2012) Feline coronavirus infections. In: Greene CE (ed) Infectious disease of the dog and cat, 4th edn. Saunders Elsevier, St. Louis, pp 92–108

2. Hartmann K (2005) Feline infectious peritonitis. Vet Clin North Am Small Anim Pract 35:39–79

3. Vennema H, Poland A, Foley J, Pedersen NC (1998) Feline infectious peritonitis viruses arise by mutation from endemic feline enteric coronaviruses. Virology 30:150–157

4. Foley JE, Pedersen NC (1996) The inheritance of susceptibility to feline infectious peritonitis in purebred catteries. Feline Pract 24:14–22

5. Pedersen NC (1976) Feline infectious peritonitis: something old, something new. Feline Pract 6:42–51

6. Sparkes AH, Gruffydd-Jones TJ, Howard PE, Harbour DA (1992) Coronavirus serology in healthy pedigree cats. Vet Rec 131:35–36

7. Addie D, Belák S, Boucraut-Baralon C et al (2009) Feline infectious peritonitis. ABCD guidelines on prevention and management. J Feline Med Surg 11:594–604

8. Herrewegh AAPM, Smeenk I, Horzinek MC, Rottier PJ, de Groot RJ (1998) Feline coronavirus type II strains 79-1683 and 79-1146 originate from a double recombination between feline coronavirus type I and canine coronavirus. J Virol 72:4508–4514

9. Vennema H, Poland A, Hawkins KF, Pedersen NC (1995) A comparison of the genomes of FECVs and FIPVs and what they tell us about the relationships between feline coronaviruses and their evolution. Feline Pract 23:40–44

10. Terada Y, Matsui N, Noguchi K et al (2014) Emergence of pathogenic coronaviruses in cats by homologous recombination between feline and canine coronaviruses. PLoS One 9:e106534

11. Benetka V, Kubber-Heiss A, Kolodziejek J et al (2004) Prevalence of feline coronavirus types I and II in cats with histopathologically verified feline infectious peritonitis. Vet Microbiol 99:31–42

12. Kummrow M, Meli ML, Haessig M et al (2005) Feline coronavirus serotypes 1 and 2: seroprevalence and association with disease in Switzerland. Clin Diagn Lab Immunol 12:1209–1215

13. Lin CN, Su BL, Wang CH et al (2009) Genetic diversity and correlation with feline infectious peritonitis of feline coronavirus type I and II: 5-year study in Taiwan. Vet Microbiol 136:233–239

14. Soma T, Wada M, Taharaguchi S, Tajima T (2013) Detection of ascitic feline coronavirus RNA from cats with clinically suspected feline infectious peritonitis. J Vet Med Sci 75:1389–1392

15. Sparkes AH, Gruffydd-Jones TJ, Harbour DA (1994) An appraisal of the value of laboratory tests in the diagnosis of feline infectious peritonitis. J Am Anim Hosp Assoc 30:345–350

16. Hartmann K, Binder C, Hirschberger J et al (2003) Comparison of different tests to diagnose feline infectious peritonitis. J Vet Intern Med 17:781–790

17. Herrewegh AAPM, de Groot RJ, Cepica A et al (1995) Detection of feline coronavirus RNA in feces, tissues, and body fluids of naturally infected cats by reverse transcriptase PCR. J Clin Microbiol 33:684–689

18. Soma T, Kawashima S, Osada H, Ishii H (2010) Diagnostic value of feline coronavirus PCR testing in clinical cases. J Environ Dis 19:1–7

19. Kennedy MA, Millsaps BRK, Potgieter BLND (1998) Correlation of genomic detection of feline coronavirus with various diagnostic assays for feline infectious peritonitis. J Vet Diagn Invest 10:93–97

20. Foley JE, Lapointe JM, Koblik P, Poland A, Pedersen NC (1998) Diagnostic features of clinical neurologic feline infectious peritonitis. J Vet Intern Med 12:415–423

21. Doenges SJ, Weber K, Dorsch R, et al Detection of feline coronavirus in cerebrospinal fluid for diagnosis of feline infectious peritonitis in cats with and without neurological signs. J Feline Med Surg Mar 3. pii: 1098612X15574757. [Epub ahead of print]

22. Fehr D, Bolla S, Herrewegh AA, Horzinek MC, Lutz H (1996) Detection of feline coronavirus using RT-PCR: basis for the study of the pathogenesis of feline infectious peritonitis (FIP). Schweiz Arch Tierheilkd 138:74–79

23. Gunn-Moore DA, Gruffydd-Jones TJ, Harbour DA (1998) Detection of feline coronaviruses by culture and reverse transcriptase-polymerase chain reaction of blood samples from healthy cats and cats with clinical feline infectious peritonitis. Vet Microbiol 62:193–205

24. Can-Sahna K, Soydal Ataseven V, Pinar D, Oğuzoğlu TC (2007) The detection of feline coronaviruses in blood samples from cats by mRNA RT-PCR. J Feline Med Surg 9:369–372

25. Herrewegh AA, Mähler M, Hedrich HJ et al (1997) Persistence and evolution of feline coronavirus in a closed cat-breeding colony. Virology 234:349–363

26. Sharif S, Arshad SS, Hair-Bejo M et al (2010) Diagnostic methods for feline coronavirus: a review. Vet Med Int 2010, 809480

27. Simons FA, Vennema H, Rofina JE et al (2005) A mRNA PCR for the diagnosis of feline infectious peritonitis. J Virol Methods 124:111–116

28. Pedersen NC, Eckstrand C, Liu H, Leutenegger C, Murphy B (2015) Levels of feline infectious peritonitis virus in blood, effusions, and various tissues and the role of lymphopenia in disease outcome following experimental infection. Vet Microbiol 175:157–166

29. Li X, Scott FW (1994) Detection of feline coronaviruses in cell cultures and in fresh and fixed feline tissues using polymerase chain reaction. Vet Microbiol 42(65–77):1994

30. Sharif S, Arshad SS, Hair-Bejo M et al (2011) Evaluation of feline coronavirus viraemia in clinically healthy and ill cats with feline infectious peritonitis. J Anim Vet Adv 10:18–22

31. Addie DD, Schaap IAT, Nicolson L, Jarrett O (2003) Persistence and transmission of natural type I feline coronavirus infection. J Gen Virol 84:2735–2744

Chapter 16

Genotype-Specific Detection of Ferret Coronavirus by Conventional and Real-Time Reverse Transcription Polymerase Chain Reaction

Annabel G. Wise, Matti Kiupel, and Roger K. Maes

Abstract

Ferret coronavirus is associated with two disease presentations in ferrets, namely, epizootic catarrhal enteritis and a feline infectious peritonitis (FIP)-like systemic disease. In this chapter, we describe conventional and real-time one-step reverse transcription polymerase chain reaction assays that are routinely used in our laboratory to detect either genotype 1 or genotype 2 ferret coronavirus in clinical specimens. These assays were designed based upon the conserved spike gene sequence difference found between three strains of ferret systemic coronavirus and three strains of ferret enteric coronavirus. Recent literature evidence indicates that pathotype is not associated with a specific genotype, and therefore, it is important to test for both genotypes either in enteric or systemic disease.

Key words Ferret coronavirus, Conventional RT-PCR, Real-time RT-PCR, Molecular diagnostic assay

1 Introduction

Epizootic catarrhal enteritis (ECE), an enteric disease of domestic ferrets was first described in the USA in 1993 [1]. Clinically, the disease is characterized by a foul-smelling bright green diarrhea with high mucus content, lethargy, anorexia, and vomiting. Morbidity approaches 100 %, but mortality is usually below 5 %, with juvenile ferrets often developing only mild disease. ECE was found to be associated with an alphacoronavirus, designated ferret enteric coronavirus (FRECV) [2]. This disease or the enteric coronavirus agent associated with it has since spread in the USA and other countries worldwide [3–5]. Close to a decade after the recognition of ECE, a systemic disease, characterized by feline infectious peritonitis (FIP)-like clinical signs and lesions, began to emerge in ferrets across the USA and Europe [6–9]. Clinical findings include anorexia, weight loss, diarrhea and the presence of

Leyi Wang (ed.), *Animal Coronaviruses*, Springer Protocols Handbooks,
DOI 10.1007/978-1-4939-3414-0_16, © Springer Science+Business Media New York 2016

large palpable intra-abdominal masses. A marked resemblance to FIP is the gross observation of widespread whitish nodules on serosal surfaces and within the parenchyma of abdominal and thoracic organs. A systemic pyogranulomatous inflammation is the consistent histologic lesion observed in the affected organs, reminiscent of FIP. The agent associated with this disease, was found to be another alphacoronavirus, designated, ferret systemic coronavirus or FRSCV, and is most closely related to FRECV [6, 10]. The disease continues to spread worldwide with more recent reports from the UK, France and Japan [11–14].

Comparative sequence analysis of the distal one-third of the genomes of one FRSCV and one FRECV strain [10] showed that these two viruses share at least 96 % nucleotide sequence identities in the membrane, nucleocapsid and non-structural protein genes, ORFs 3 and 7b. However, their spike (S) proteins showed only 79.6 % amino acid sequence identity. This allowed the development of two S genotype-specific conventional [10], as well as real-time RT-PCR assays [15] for routine detection of these viruses in our laboratory. Limited preliminary data have shown that genotype 1 (FRSCV-like) ferret coronaviruses were found associated with the systemic type of illness while genotype 2 (FRECV-like) ferret coronaviruses were detected in cases of ECE [10]. Recent literature evidence indicates that there is no association between the S genotype and virus pathotype [4, 5]. The differentiating genotype-specific RT-PCR assays were recently used in a study that determined the prevalence of coronavirus among domestic ferrets in Japan [5]. The investigators noted that the majority of ferrets that were shedding the genotype 1 ferret coronavirus in feces were not ill with the systemic disease and that some were even asymptomatic. In the Netherlands, partial spike gene sequence analysis reported by Provacia et al. [4] showed that genotype 1 ferret coronavirus strains were also found present in feces of asymptomatic ferrets. These findings bring to mind the "in vivo mutation" theory proposed by Chang et al. [16] and Pedersen [17] for FIP-inducing feline coronavirus strains. It may well be the case for ferret coronaviruses that the virus commonly found in normal feces may just be the "precursor" to a more pathogenic strain. Wise et al. [10] noted the presence of a truncated 3c-like protein gene in two out of three genotype 1 strains identified in ferrets with systemic disease, reminiscent of the 3c gene mutations identified in FIP viruses in cats [16–18].

Polymerase chain reaction (PCR) is a method to amplify a fragment of double-stranded DNA to millions of copies, based upon repeated cycles of double-stranded DNA template denaturation, primer annealing and elongation. A primer is a short single-stranded DNA sequence, also called an oligonucleotide, that "primes" the reaction at the appropriate annealing temperature by binding to the complementary sequence of the denatured DNA target. Using the deoxyribonucleotides (dNTPs) in the reaction, the Taq polymerase enzyme then catalyzes the polymerization of nucleotides to polynucleotides beginning at the 3′ end of the primer in the elongation step. Reverse transcription polymerase chain reaction (RT-PCR) is used when the original target template is RNA, such that the RNA is first reverse-transcribed into "copy DNA," or cDNA, by the reverse transcriptase enzyme. The cDNA is then amplified in the PCR step. Conventional PCR/RT-PCR [19–22] requires the visualization of the amplified DNA or the PCR product, in an agarose gel matrix submerged in buffer through the process of electrophoresis. Electrophoresis subjects the PCR product to an electric current flow in the buffer that causes the DNA to migrate through the gel matrix according to its molecular weight. The PCR product is stained with an intercalating dye that fluoresces upon exposure to UV light, enabling its visualization alongside a DNA size marker ladder.

In real-time PCR/RT-PCR [19–22], the amplified DNA or the amplicon, is detected and recorded in "real-time" during the assay itself. With a hydrolysis probe-based real-time PCR, also called a "Taqman"-probe based assay, the amplification of DNA in every cycle results to a steady buildup of fluorescence signal in the reaction that can be detected using a specialized thermocycler with a built-in real-time nucleic acid detection system (e.g., Cepheid SmartCycler system). The probe, an essential component of the reaction mix, is a synthetic oligonucleotide with a sequence complementary to the target DNA flanked by the primers. The probe is labeled at its 5′ end with a fluorescent reporter dye (e.g., FAM) and with a fluorescence quencher (e.g., BHQ-1) at its 3′ end. There is no fluorescent signal emitted as long as the probe remains intact. In the presence of the specific target DNA in the reaction, after the primers and probe anneal to their complementary sequence, polymerization takes place in the elongation phase of the PCR cycle, during which the probe is degraded via the 5′ exonuclease activity of the Taq DNA polymerase. Probe degradation leads to the release of the reporter dye from the probe and from its proximity to the quencher molecule, resulting to the accumulation of fluorescence signal in the reaction mix at every PCR cycle.

2 Materials

2.1 RNA Extraction

1. QIAGEN RNeasy Mini Kit.
2. β-mercaptoethanol (β-ME).
3. Ethanol (EtOH), 96–100 % grade.
4. 70 % EtOH (prepared by adding three parts molecular grade water to seven parts 100 % EtOH).
5. RNase/DNase-free water (molecular grade water).

6. Clinical samples: feces; tissues.

7. 0.1 M phosphate buffered saline (PBS).

8. Micropipettes, sterile and RNAse-free pipette tips (filtered tips are preferable), autoclaved/sterile microcentrifuge tubes (1.5–2 ml capacity), microcentrifuge tube rack.

9. Disposable gloves; protective clothing and eyewear.

2.2 One-Step Reverse Transcription Polymerase Chain Reaction

1. QIAGEN OneStep RT-PCR Kit.

   Components of the kit:

   (a) 5× OneStep RT-PCR Buffer.

   (b) dNTP Mix (containing 10 mM of each dNTP).

   (c) OneStep RT-PCR Enzyme Mix (contains HotStarTaq DNA Polymerase and Omniscript and Sensiscript reverse transcriptases).

   (d) RNase/DNase-free water.

2. 25 mM $MgCl_2$ solution.

3. Genotype 1-specific (G1) primers (*see* **Note 1**).

   (a) 20 µM G1 forward primer, 5′-CTGGTGTTTGTGCAAC ATCTAC-3′.

   (b) 20 µM G1 reverse primer, 5′-TCTATTTGCACAAAAT CAGACA-3′,

4. Genotype 2-specific (G2) primers (*see* **Note 1**).

   (a) 20 µM G2 forward primer, 5′-GGCATTTGTTTTGATA ACGTTG-3′.

   (b) 20 µM G2 reverse primer, 5′-CTATTAATTCGCACGAA ATCTGC-3′.

5. Known genotype 1 or 2 ferret coronavirus positive RNA (positive control).

6. RNase/DNase-free water (negative control).

7. Micropipettes, filtered tips, sterile RNAse-free microcentrifuge tubes, 0.2 ml PCR tubes, and PCR tube rack.

8. PCR tube mini-centrifuge.

9. Thermocycler (ABI 2720, Applied Biosystems).

2.3 Agarose Gel Electrophoresis

1. 50× TAE (Tris–acetate–EDTA) buffer.

2. Agarose powder.

3. 100 bp DNA Ladder (New England Biolabs).

4. 6× gel loading buffer (this comes with the DNA ladder).

5. Ethidium bromide, 10 mg/ml.

6. Gel casting tray (for 100 ml gel volume) and comb (10-slot comb) (*see* **Note 2**).

7. Agarose gel electrophoresis apparatus.

8. Power supply.

9. UV light box/transilluminator; UV protective face shield.

10. Gel photography equipment.

2.4 Taqman Probe-based One-Step Real-Time (rt) RT-PCR

1. AgPath ID One-Step RT-PCR Kit (Applied Biosystems, ThermoFisher).

2. Genotype 1-specific (G1rt) primers and probe (*see* **Notes 1** and **3**).

   (a) 20 μM G1rt forward primer, 5′-GATGTGTCGTTGACK TTRTT-3′.

   (b) 20 μM G1rt reverse primer, 5′-TGGTGCAGCTTTCTA TTTGC-3′.

   (c) 6 μM G1rt probe, 5′-(FAM)ACRCCGCGTACAATGTAC GAACC(BHQ-1)-3′ (FAM, 6-carboxy-fluorescein; BHQ-1, blackhole quencher 1).

3. Genotype 2-specific (G2rt) primers and probe (*see* **Notes 1, 4** and **5**).

   (a) 20 μM G2rt forward primer, 5′-GGCATTTGTTTTG ATAACGTTG-3′.

   (b) 20 μM G2rt reverse primer, 5′-CTATTAATTCGCACGA AATCTGC-3′.

   (c) 10 μM G2rt probe, 5′-(FAM)CTCATACATAGTAC GTG(MGB-NFQ)-3′ (FAM, 6-carboxy-fluorescein; MGB-NFQ, minor-groove binding probe-nonfluorescent quencher).

4. Real-time PCR instrument (SmartCycler II, by Cepheid, Inc.); computer and software.

5. SmartCycler PCR reaction tubes, SmartCycler reaction tube rack, Smart Tube benchtop centrifuge.

3 Methods

3.1 RNA Extraction

1. Reconstituting reagents in a new QIAGEN RNeasy Mini Kit (*see* **Note 6**).

   (a) Add 10 μl of β-ME (*see* **Note 7**) for every 10 ml of buffer RLT (lysis buffer) (*see* **Note 8**).

   This lysis buffer is stable at room temperature for 1 month after the addition of β-ME.

(b) Add 4 volumes of ethanol to the new bottle of RPE buffer (supplied as a concentrate), according to the manufacturer's instructions as indicated on the bottle to obtain a working solution.

2. Sample preparation (*see* **Note 9**):

(a) Prepare ~10 % fecal homogenate by diluting feces in 0.1 M PBS. Clarify the sample by centrifuging for 5 min at 2500 rpm (~580 rcf for a 24-well microcentrifuge (e.g. Eppendorf Centrifuge 5417C)).

(b) For tissues, prepare ~10 % tissue homogenate in 0.1 M PBS (*see* **Note 10**).

3. Pipet 140 μl of sample into a microcentrifuge tube.

4. Add 560 μl of buffer RLT with β-ME to the sample. Mix gently by pipetting.

5. Add 700 μl of 70 % EtOH to the lysed sample. Mix gently by pipetting.

6. Transfer 700 μl of the sample solution to an RNeasy mini column supplied with a 2-ml filtrate collection tube.

7. Close the column and centrifuge for 30 s at 10,000 rpm. Discard the filtrate and reuse the collection tube in **step 8**.

8. Transfer the remaining sample solution (~700 μl) to the same RNeasy mini column and centrifuge for 30 s at 10,000 rpm. Discard the filtrate and reuse the collection tube in **step 9**.

9. Add 700 μl of buffer RW1 (*see* **Note 11**) to the RNeasy mini column. Close the column and centrifuge for 30 s at 10,000 rpm. Discard the filtrate and the collection tube.

10. Place the RNeasy mini column into a new 2 ml collection tube. Add 500 μl of buffer RPE (previously reconstituted with EtOH) to the column for a first wash. Close the column and centrifuge the column for 30 s at 10,000 rpm. Discard the filtrate and reuse the collection tube in **step 11**.

11. Add another 500 μl of buffer RPE to the RNeasy column for the second wash. Close the column and centrifuge for 2 min at 10,000 rpm. Discard the filtrate and collection tube.

12. Place the RNeasy mini column with the cap closed into a new 2 ml collection tube. Dry spin the column for 1 min at 14,000 rpm. Residual RPE buffer will be removed from the column (*see* **Note 12**). Discard the collection tube.

13. To elute the RNA, place the RNeasy mini column into a new microcentrifuge tube. Pipet 100 μl of RNase/DNase-free water into the column close to the silica-gel membrane. Close the column, let stand for 1 min at room temperature, then centrifuge for 1 min at 10,000 rpm. Discard the column.

14. Put the microcentrifuge tube with the extracted RNA on ice (*see* **Note 13**). The RNA sample is now ready to be tested.

Store the RNA in refrigeration temperature if testing within 24 h. Store it in −20 or −80 °C if testing will be delayed for more than 24 h.

3.2 One-Step
RT-PCR Assay

1. Working in a designated "clean" PCR station (*see* **Note 14**), thaw the OneStep RT-PCR kit reagents and working stock primers on ice. In a sterile microcentrifuge tube, prepare the master mix for the number of reactions needed per genotype test according to Tables 1 and 2. Total number of reactions (N) equals the number of samples to be tested, plus two more for positive and negative controls, then add to this subtotal 10 % more reactions for overage allowance.

Table 1
Components of RT-PCR master mix (genotype 1-specific)

Master mix reagent	Volume per reaction (μl)	Volume for N reactions (μl)	Final concentration
5× QIAGEN OneStep RT-PCR buffer	10	$10 \times N$	1×
dNTP mix	2	$2 \times N$	0.4 mM
25 mM MgCl$_2$	2.5	$2.5 \times N$	1.25 mM
G1 forward primer, 20 μM	1.25	$1.25 \times N$	0.5 μM
G1 reverse primer, 20 μM	1.25	$1.25 \times N$	0.5 μM
QIAGEN OneStep Enzyme Mix	2	$2 \times N$	–
RNase-free water	33	$33 \times N$	–
Total	45		

Table 2
Components of RT-PCR master mix (genotype 2-specific)

Master mix reagent	Volume per reaction (μl)	Volume for N reactions (μl)	Final concentration
5× QIAGEN OneStep RT-PCR buffer	10	$10 \times N$	1×
dNTP mix	2	$2 \times N$	0.4 mM
25 mM MgCl$_2$	2.5	$2.5 \times N$	1.25 mM
G2 forward primer, 20 μM	1.25	$1.25 \times N$	0.5 μM
G2 reverse primer, 20 μM	1.25	$1.25 \times N$	0.5 μM
QIAGEN OneStep RT-PCR Enzyme Mix	2	$2 \times N$	–
RNase-free water	33	$33 \times N$	–
Total	45		

2. Mix the contents of the tube by pipetting gently. Keep the master mix tube on ice.

3. Dispense 45 μl of master mix to each 0.2 μl PCR tube. For the negative control, add 5 μl of sterile RNase/DNase-free water to the last PCR tube, then close the tube (*see* **Note 15**).

4. Transfer to the template addition area/hood. Keeping a record of the order of samples and controls, add 5 μl of each sample RNA (template) to a PCR tube, closing the tube cap after each template addition.

5. Add 5 μl of positive control RNA (known positive genotype 1 or 2 ferret coronavirus RNA) to the last open tube (*see* **Note 16**). Close the cap.

6. Centrifuge the tubes briefly.

7. Place the tubes in the thermocycler and run the RT-PCR reaction according to the cycling protocol shown in Table 3.

8. When the run is completed, analyze the PCR products by agarose gel electrophoresis. The products may be kept in the refrigerator or frozen for short-term holding.

3.3 Agarose Gel Electrophoresis

1. Preparing 1 l (1000 ml) of 1× TAE buffer from a 50× TAE stock solution:

    (a) Pour 20 ml of 50× concentrated TAE buffer into a 1 l graduated cylinder.

    (b) Fill the cylinder with deionized water up to the 1 l line, making a 1× final concentration of TAE buffer.

2. Preparing a working stock solution of 100 bp DNA ladder with pre-added loading dye:

Table 3
Cycling conditions for RT-PCR

Step	Temperature (°C)	Time
1. Reverse transcription	50	30 min
2. Heat activation/inactivation	95	15 min
3. PCR cycling (40 cycles)		
Denaturation	94	30 s
Annealing	55	30 s
Extension	72	30 s
4. Final Extension	72	7 min
5. Hold	4	∞

(a) To a new tube of 100 bp DNA ladder, add 500 μl DNase-free water and 80 μl of the 6× loading dye/buffer.

(b) Mix evenly by gently pipetting up and down.

3. Preparing a 2 % agarose gel:

(a) Assemble the gel-casting tray on the gel-casting rack. Using a level indicator, make sure it is level. Position the gel comb on the tray slots.

(b) Weigh 2 g of agarose powder on a clean weighing paper or boat. In a 250 ml Erlenmeyer flask, pour the 2 g agarose powder then add 100 ml of 1× TAE buffer. Swirl the flask gently to mix.

(c) Microwave the flask on high for about 2 min or until the agarose is completely melted, with the solution bubbling and turning clear/transparent (see **Note 17**).

(d) After microwaving, add 5 μl of the ethidium bromide solution to the melted agarose. Grasping the flask with a heat-protective mitten, swirl the flask gently until the ethidium bromide is evenly distributed in the solution (see **Note 18**).

(e) Pour the gel solution into the gel tray and let stand for at least 45 min in room temperature or until the gel becomes solidified. The gel will have a thickness of about 0.8 cm.

4. Remove the gel tray with the casted 2 % gel from the casting rack. Gently lift the comb out of the gel (see **Note 19**).

5. Place the gel tray onto the electrophoresis tank at the correct orientation (the top of the gel next to the negative lead or cathode [black]). Pour enough 1× TAE buffer into the tank buffer chamber to submerge the gel with about 2–3 mm of buffer above the surface of the gel.

6. Add 10 μl of the 6× gel loading dye to the 50 μl PCR product in each tube. Mix evenly by gentle pipetting.

7. In the first well of the gel, load 30 μl of the 100 bp DNA ladder working stock solution.

8. Load 50 μl of each PCR product with the dye in the succeeding wells (see **Note 20**).

9. Close the lid of the tank and connect the color-coded wires/leads to the appropriate sockets of the power supply and the gel tank (black to black, red to red). DNA migrates toward the positive lead or anode (red).

10. Turn on the power supply. Set the voltage output to 100 V. Run for approximately 45 min to 1 h checking the dye level for adequate product migration time (see **Note 21**).

11. When DNA migration is complete, turn off the power supply. Unplug the leads from the gel tank, lift the cover and remove the gel tray.

12. Set the gel on top of the UV transilluminator. Turn off the room light.

13. While wearing a UV protective face shield, turn the UV light on to visualize the gel.

14. The expected product sizes are: 157 bp for genotype 1 and 146 bp for genotype 2 ferret coronavirus (Fig. 1a, b).

15. Document the results with the photo-documentation instrument. Turn the UV light off when finished.

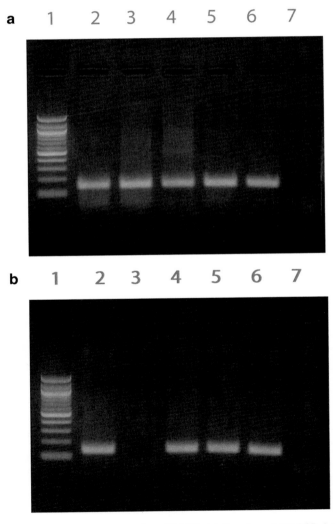

Fig. 1 Conventional ferret coronavirus RT-PCR. (a) Genotype 1 RT-PCR. Lanes: 1, 100 bp DNA ladder; 2–5, positive samples; 6, positive control (157 bp); 7, negative control. (b) Genotype 2 RT-PCR. Lanes: 1, 100 bp DNA ladder; 2, 4, and 5, positive samples; 3, negative sample; 6, positive control (146 bp); 7, negative control

3.4 Taqman Probe-Based One-Step Real-Time RT-PCR

1. Turn on the computer and the SmartCycler machine. The SmartCycler block will display a lighted "0" at the bottom left corner of the top surface of the instrument.

2. Click on the SmartCycler software icon to start the program. If using only one SmartCycler block, it will be designated as block "A". The lighted "0" will switch to the letter designation (*see* **Note 22**). This confirms that the computer has established connection with the instrument.

3. Click "Define Graphs" located at the toolbar on the top of the screen (*see* **Note 23**).

   (a) Select "FAM" under the Graph list, then select or check the box for the following options: Check "Automatically added to new Runs"; for "Graph Type" select Optics; for "Channels" select Ch 1; under "Show" check Primary Curve, Threshold (Horizontal) and Threshold Crossings (Vertical); for "Axes" select Fluorescence vs. Cycle. Click "Save Graph".

   (b) Select "Temperature" under the Graph list. Then select or check the box for "Sample Temperature". Check "Automatically added to new Runs". Click "Save Graph".

4. Click "Define Protocols" located in the tool bar at the top of the screen. Click "New Protocol" at the bottom of the screen, then type a "Protocol Name" (e.g., Ferret Coronavirus S Genotyping) and enter the cycling protocol parameters according to Table 4. Save the protocol.

5. Click "Create a Run".

Table 4
Cycling conditions for real-time RT-PCR

Step	Temperature (°C)	Time	Optics
[a]1. Reverse transcription	45	10 min	Off
[a]2. Heat activation/inactivation	95	15 min	Off
3. PCR cycling (45 cycles)			
[b]Denaturation	94	10 s	Off
[b]Annealing	55	30 s	On
[b]Extension	72	10 s	Off

[a]In defining a protocol in the SmartCycler, enter these steps as "Stage 1 with 2-Temperature Cycle". Enter "1.6" under Deg/Sec column
[b]In defining a protocol in the SmartCycler, enter these steps as "Stage 2 with 3-Temperature Cycle". Enter "1.6" under Deg/Sec column

6. Assign a "Run Name".

7. Leave the Dye Set at the default setting, "FCTC25."

8. Click "Select Graphs" at the bottom of the screen. Under "All Graphs" on the left side of the screen, highlight "FAM" and "Temperature", then click the right-pointing arrow to transfer these graphs under "Selected Graphs" on the right. Click "OK". Unused graphs under "Selected Graphs", if present, may be deselected by highlighting the graphs then clicking the left-pointing arrow.

9. For Channel/Dye settings, leave FAM at the default Usage setting, "Assay". All other dyes/fluorophores (Cy3, TxR, and Cy5) may be set to "Unused" (*see* **Note 24**).

10. For Analysis Settings, set "Bkgnd Max Cycle" (background maximum cycle) at 28 and "Manual Thresh Fluor Units" (manual threshold fluorescence units) at 25. Leave the rest of the analysis settings at default.

11. Click "Add Remove Sites". Select the appropriate protocol from the protocol list. Select the "sites" or "wells" to be used (e.g., A1, A2, A3) depending on the number of samples to be run, plus two more sites for the positive and the negative controls.

12. Click the arrowhead symbol to add the sites to the selections column on the right. Click the "OK" button.

13. Enter the Sample IDs in the table.

14. Prepare the RT-PCR master mix according to Tables 5 or 6.

15. On a chilled SmartCycler reaction tube rack (*see* **Note 25**), put the appropriate number of SmartCycler reaction tubes needed

Table 5
Components of real-time RT-PCR master mix (genotype 1-specific)

Master mix reagent	Volume per reaction (µl)	Volume for N reactions (µl)	Final concentration
2× AgPath ID One-Step RT-PCR buffer	12.5	$12.5 \times N$	1×
Enhancer	1.67	$1.67 \times N$	–
G1rt forward primer, 20 µM	0.62	$0.62 \times N$	0.5 µM
G1rt reverse primer, 20 µM	0.62	$0.62 \times N$	0.5 µM
G1rt probe, 6 µM	0.5	$0.5 \times N$	120 nM
AgPath ID One-Step RT-PCR enzyme mix 1 µl	1	$1 \times N$	
RNase-free water	0.09	$0.09 \times N$	–
Total	17		

Table 6
Components of real-time RT-PCR master mix (genotype 2-specific)

Master mix reagent	Volume per reaction (µl)	Volume for *N* reactions (µl)	Final concentration
2× AgPath ID One-Step RT-PCR buffer	12.5	$12.5 \times N$	1×
Enhancer	1.67	$1.67 \times N$	–
G2rt forward primer, 20 µM	0.62	$0.62 \times N$	0.5 µM
G2rt reverse primer, 20 µM	0.62	$0.62 \times N$	0.5 µM
G2rt probe, 10 µM	0.5	$0.5 \times N$	200 nM
AgPath ID One-Step RT-PCR enzyme mix	1	$1 \times N$	–
RNase-free water	0.09	$0.09 \times N$	–
Total	17		

for the run. Number each tube at the cap surface to keep track of the sample order.

16. Dispense 17 µl of master mix into each tube. Add 8 µl of sample RNA, positive control RNA, and RNAse-free water (no template control) into the appropriate tube, then cap each tube tightly.

17. Spin the tubes for 3–5 s using the Smart Tube mini-centrifuge.

18. Load the tubes in the pre-selected SmartCycler sites/wells, then securely close the top cover of each site.

19. Click "Start Run". Run-time is approximately 1 h and 40 min.

20. When the run is finished, the Results Table will show for each Site ID whether the sample is "positive" or "negative". Positive samples, including the positive control, will have a FAM Ct (cycle threshold) > 0. Negative samples, including the negative control, will have a FAM Ct = 0.00 (*see* **Note 26**).

21. These tabulated results should be confirmed by viewing the amplification curve, also known as growth curve, for each sample and control, by selecting "FAM" under the "Views" pane. A sample is truly positive when the plot of its fluorescence vs. cycle number produces a sigmoidal shaped amplification curve as it crosses the threshold setting and continues to generate increasing fluorescent signal until it plateaus or reaches the last cycle (Fig. 2). The amplification graph of a negative sample and the negative control will appear as a flat line (Fig. 2) (*see* **Note 26**).

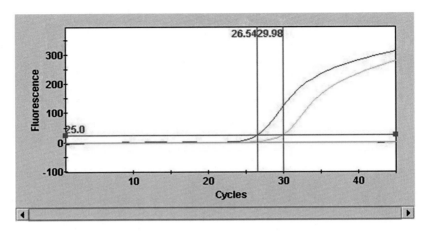

Fig. 2 Real-time PCR for ferret coronavirus genotype 1. Sigmoidal amplification curves generated by a positive sample (Ct = 29.98) and a positive control (Ct = 26.54). Manual threshold fluorescence is set at "25", indicated by the *red horizontal line*. The negative control appears as a *flat green line* at the "0" fluorescence level

4 Notes

1. Commercially ordered primers come in a dried down state. The amount of the primer in nanomoles (nanomoles × 1000 = picomoles) is stated on the tube. For each new primer tube, divide the number of picomoles (pmol) by 200 pmol/μl. The number derived equals the amount of sterile 1× TE (Tris EDTA) buffer or RNAse/DNAse-free water, in microliters, to be added to the tube to obtain a 10× primer stock of 200 μM concentration. To obtain a 20 μM 1× working primer stock, dilute (1:10) 5 μl of the 10× stock in 45 μl of RNAse/DNAse-free water. Store 10× primer stocks and 1× working stocks in –20 °C or colder.

2. A smaller gel size (50 ml) may be used with the appropriate comb size and electrophoresis tank. Adjust amount of agarose powder and TAE buffer volumes in **step** 3 of Sect. 3.3, accordingly.

3. A commercially ordered FAM/BHQ-1 labeled probe comes in a dried down state. The amount of probe in nanomoles (nanomoles × 1000 = picomoles) is stated on the tube. Divide the number of picomoles by 120 pmol/μl. The number derived equals the amount of sterile 1× TE buffer, in microliters, to be added to the tube to obtain a 20× probe stock. To obtain a 6 μM 1× working probe stock, dilute (1:20) 5 μl of the 20× stock in 95 μl of RNAse/DNAse-free water. Store probe stocks in amber-colored tubes (probes are light-sensitive) at –20 °C or colder. Avoid freeze-thawing working probe stocks more than four times to prevent degradation of the probe.

4. A MGB/NFQ-labeled probe can be ordered from ThermoFisher Scientific and is supplied as a 100 μM solution. This is the 10× probe stock. To obtain a 10 μM 1× working probe stock, dilute 5 μl of the 10× stock solution in 45 μl of RNAse/DNAse-free water. Use amber-colored tubes for the working stocks and store probes at –20 °C or colder.

5. G2 rt primers have the same sequences as the G2 primers for conventional RT-PCR.

6. Refer to the RNeasy Mini Handbook for description of the RNeasy principle/technology, additional chemical safety information (e.g., how to obtain material safety data sheets online), troubleshooting tips, and general remarks on handling RNA.

7. β-ME is a toxic chemical that must be dispensed in a chemical fume hood. Always handle with gloves, protective clothing and eyewear (personal protective gear).

8. Buffer RLT contains guanidine thiocyanate. It is harmful by inhalation, in contact with skin, and if swallowed.

9. When handling fresh animal tissues and feces, personal protective gear must be worn at all times and work must take place in Biosafety Level (BSL) 2 containment using a BSL 2 hood with the HEPA-filter blower on. The blower may be turned off once the specimens are inactivated in the RLT lysis buffer.

10. For animals exhibiting FIP-like lesions, collect sections of grossly affected tissues (i.e., mesenteric adipose tissue and lymph nodes, lung, liver, and spleen). Tissue homogenization is optimally performed by rapid agitation in the presence of a bead or beads using a laboratory mixer mill. Alternatively (if a mixer mill is not available), 25 mg of tissue can be directly disrupted and homogenized in 750 μl of buffer RLT with β-ME in a microcentrifuge tube using a disposable RNAse-free pestle. The tube is then centrifuged for 5 min at 5000 rpm (~2300 rcf for a 24-well microcentrifuge (i.e. Eppendorf Centrifuge 5417 C) to clarify the lysate. Transfer 700 μl of the lysate into a fresh tube, then proceed directly to **step** 5 (addition of 70 % EtOH) to continue with the RNA extraction.

11. Buffer RW1 contains ethanol and therefore is flammable.

12. Removal of residual RPE buffer in this step is crucial. The wash buffer contains EtOH which is inhibitory to PCR.

13. Holding RNA samples at 4 °C or below prior to running the RT-PCR is very important to keep its integrity. This minimizes the chance of any trace contamination with ribonucleases (RNase enzymes) in the sample to be active and degrade the RNA.

14. To minimize exposure of a PCR reaction to RNA/DNA contamination that lead to false positives, it is optimal to designate a "clean" room where master mixes can be prepared separate

from where nucleic acids are extracted and PCR templates added. Additionally designate "clean" pipettes for use solely for master mix preparation and dispensing, and negative control addition.

15. The purpose of the negative control is to monitor the integrity of the master mix, ascertaining that it remains free of contaminating positive PCR template (no amplicon observed in the gel) for the run to be valid.

16. It is best to use a positive control RNA template diluted sufficiently to a working concentration that produces only a moderately strong band/amplicon in the gel. This will minimize the production of large amounts of positive PCR products that build up over time in the environment and often lead to PCR contamination.

17. Take care that the agarose solution does not boil over while melting it in the microwave. To prevent this from occurring, the microwave should be turned off immediately as bubbling starts to occur, the flask taken out and swirled for even mixing of the solution, then heated again in the microwave until the agarose is completely melted. Protective mitts must always be used when handling the flask with the heated/melted agarose.

18. Ethidium bromide is a mutagenic substance. Always wear personal protective gear when working with this chemical.

19. Before pulling out the combs, make sure that the agarose gel is already fully set. The gel at the bottom of the wells will get torn off as the comb is lifted out if the gel is not yet fully set. Prior to use, always check that the gel is intact at the bottom of every well. A hole in the bottom of the well will cause the loaded PCR product to leak out.

20. If using gel combs with smaller teeth, decrease the amount of PCR product + loading dye to be applied, accordingly, to each well, taking care that the product does not overflow out of the well. Overflow will lead to contamination of the neighboring well which may lead to false positives.

21. Bromophenol blue, a common loading dye, migrates at a rate similar to that of a 300 bp DNA fragment.

22. Each SmartCycler II processing block or unit has 16 sites or wells. Each site or well is an independently controlled and programmable I-CORE (Intelligent Cooling/Heating Optical Reaction) module. Up to six blocks may be daisy-chained together and operated with a single computer, mimicking a 96-well reaction set-up. Each block gets designated a letter, from "A" to "F", in a 6-block set-up.

23. Alternatively, a graph may be created from scratch by clicking "New Graph" at the bottom of the screen, assigning a name to the graph (e.g., FAM Amp curve), then selecting the options

on the right depending on the purpose of the graph, then click "Save Graph".

24. Changing the "Usage" setting of the nonrelevant dyes, Cy3, TxR, and Cy5, from "Assay" to "Unused" will remove the data columns assigned for these dyes in the Results Table, leaving results displayed only for "FAM", giving a more compact table of results.

25. To chill a SmartCycler reaction tube rack, we recommend just keeping it in the refrigerator (4 °C) and not in the freezer.

26. The Ct (cycle threshold) value is the PCR cycle number at which the fluorescence signal emitted by the generated PCR product is above background noise and crosses the manually set threshold line. The higher the amount of the starting target template in the sample, the lower the Ct value. A negative sample or control will not cross the threshold throughout the run and will have a Ct = 0. If the negative control shows a Ct > 0, this indicates that there is template contamination in the master mix, and hence the results of the run are not valid. The contamination issue should be addressed and the run repeated.

References

1. Williams BH, Kiupel M, West KH et al (2000) Coronavirus-associated epizootic catarrhal enteritis in ferrets. J Am Vet Med Assoc 217:526–530

2. Wise AG, Kiupel M, Maes RK (2006) Molecular characterization of a novel coronavirus associated with epizootic catarrhal enteritis (ECE) in ferrets. Virology 349:164–174

3. Gregori F, Catroxo MHB, Lopes VDS et al (2010) Occurrence of ferret enteric coronavirus in Brazil (preliminary report). Braz J Vet Res Anim Sci São Paulo 47:156–158

4. Provacia LBV, Smits SL, Martina BE et al (2011) Enteric coronavirus in ferrets, the Netherlands. Emerg Infect Dis 17:1570–1571

5. Terada Y, Minami S, Noguchi K et al (2014) Genetic characterization of coronaviruses from domestic ferrets, Japan. Emerg Infect Dis 20:284–287

6. Garner MM, Ramsell K, Morera N et al (2008) Clinicopathologic features of a systemic coronavirus-associated disease resembling feline infectious peritonitis in the domestic ferret (Mustelaputorius). Vet Pathol 45:236–246

7. Juan-Sallés C, Teifke N, Morera N et al (2006) Pathology and immunohistochemistry of a disease resembling feline infectious peritonitis in ferrets (Mustelaputoriusfuro). Proc Am Col Vet Pathol 84:845

8. Martinez J, Ramis AJ, Reinacher M, Perpiñán D (2006) Detection of feline infectious peritonitis virus-like antigen in ferrets. Vet Rec 158:523

9. Martinez J, Reinacher M, Perpiñán D, Ramis A (2008) Identification of group 1 coronavirus antigen in multisystemic granulomatous lesions in ferrets (Musteloputoriusfuro). J Comp Pathol 138:54–58

10. Wise AG, Kiupel M, Garner MM, Clark AK, Maes RK (2010) Comparative sequence analysis of the distal one-third of the genomes of a systemic and an enteric ferret coronavirus. Virus Res 149:42–50

11. Graham E, Lamm C, Denk D et al (2012) Systemic coronavirus-associated disease resembling feline infectious peritonitis in ferrets in the UK. Vet Rec 171:200–201

12. Linsart A, Nicolier A, Sauvaget S (2013) Unusual presentation of systemic coronavirus is in a ferret. PMCAC 48:123–128

13. Michimae Y, Mikami S, Okimoto K et al (2010) The first case of feline infectious peritonitis-like pyogranuloma in a ferret infected by coronavirus in Japan. J Toxicol Pathol 23:99–101

14. Shigemoto J, Muraoka Y, Wise AG et al (2014) Two cases of systemic coronavirus-associated disease resembling feline infectious peritonitis

in domestic ferrets in Japan. J Exot Pet Med 23:196–100

15. Wise AG, Kiupel M, Maes RK (2011) Emerging coronaviruses of ferrets. In: Abstracts of the XII International Nidovirus Symposium, Traverse City, MI, 4–9 June 2011

16. Chang HW, de Groot RJ, Egberink HF, Rottier PJ (2010) Feline infectious peritonitis: Insights into feline coronavirus pathobiogenesis and epidemiology based on genetic analysis of the viral 3c gene. J Gen Virol 91:415–420

17. Pedersen NC (2009) A review of feline enteric coronavirus infection. J Feline Med Surg 11:225–258

18. Pedersen NC, Liu H, Scarlett J et al (2012) Feline infectious peritonitis: role of the feline coronavirus 3c gene in intestinal tropism and pathogenicity based upon isolates from resident and adopted shelter cats. Virus Res 165:17–28

19. Parida MM (2008) Rapid and real-time detection technologies for emerging viruses of biomedical importance. J Biosci 33:617–628

20. Ratcliff RM, Chang G, Kok T et al (2007) Molecular diagnosis of medical viruses. Curr Issues Mol Biol 9:87–102

21. Sellon RK (2003) Update on molecular techniques for diagnostic testing of infectious disease. Vet Clin North Am Small Anim Pract 33:677–693

22. Yang S, Rothman RE (2004) PCR-based diagnostics for infectious diseases: uses, limitations, and future applications in acute-care settings. Lancet Infect Dis 4:337–348

Chapter 17

Molecular Characterization of Canine Coronavirus

Rita de Cássia Nasser Cubel Garcia

Abstract

Canine coronavirus (CCoV) is usually the cause of mild gastroenteritis in dogs and is known to have spread worldwide. In the last decade, as a consequence of the extraordinary large RNA genome, novel recombinant variants of CCoV have been found that are closely related to feline and porcine strains. Moreover highly virulent pantropic CCoV strains were recently identified in dogs. The molecular characterization of the CCoV circulating in canine population is essential for understanding viral evolution.

Key words Canine coronavirus, Enteritis, RT-PCR, Sequencing, Genotype

1 Introduction and Background

Canine coronavirus (CCoV), a common enteric pathogen of dogs, belongs to the *Coronaviridae* family, genus *Alphacoronavirus* along with feline coronavirus (FCoV) and transmissible gastroenteritis virus (TGEV); these viruses display greater than 96 % sequence identity within the replicase polyprotein gene [1, 2].

The CCoV genome is a single-stranded, positive-sense RNA of approximately 30 kb, and includes 7–10 open reading frames (ORFs). The 5′ two-thirds of the genome (ORF-1) consists of two overlapping regions (1a and 1b) that are translated in a polyprotein which is the precursor both of the viral replicase—Rep and proteases. Another one-third nucleotide sequences from the 3′ end contain smaller ORFs encoding for the structural proteins: ORF2—spike (S), ORF4—envelope (E), ORF5—membrane (M), and ORF6—nucleocapsid (N) proteins. These ORFs are interspersed with several ORFs (3a, 3b, 3c, 7a, and 7b) encoding various non-structural proteins, most of which of unknown function (Fig. 1) [2–4].

To date, CCoVs can be classified into two genotypes, CCoV-I and CCoV-II. This classification is not related to the chronologic order of the isolates but to the genetic identity between these viruses and FCoV types I and II [5].

Leyi Wang (ed.), *Animal Coronaviruses*, Springer Protocols Handbooks,
DOI 10.1007/978-1-4939-3414-0_17, © Springer Science+Business Media New York 2016

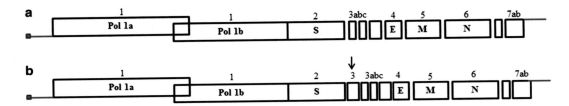

Fig. 1 Genetic structure of CCoV type II (a) and CCoV type I (b). Adapted from Pratelli, 2011. The *numbers above the bars* indicate ORFs. The *arrow* (b) indicates an intact ORF 3 downstream of the gene S, unique to CoCV-I

Genetic analysis of several CCoVs detected in pups with diarrhea in Italy revealed a number of point mutations affecting a fragment of the M gene, which has led to the designation of these atypical CCoVs as FCoV-like CCoVs, based on their similarity to the commonly circulating FCoV strains (FCoV-I). Subsequently, these viruses were designated CCoV-I (prototype—Elmo/02 strains) to discriminate them from previously identified reference viruses which were classified as CCoV-II (prototypes—Insavac-1. K378) [5–7]. In addition to the genomic differences identified in M gene, it is now known that the major differences between viruses belonging to CCoV-I and CCoV-II are primarily found within the S protein (Fig. 2) [8].

Recently, CCoV-II strain was divided in two subtypes: CCoV-IIa (classical strains) and IIb (TGEV-like strains) based on the sequence of the first 300 amino acids of the S protein: N-terminal domain-NTD region [9, 10]. CCoV-IIb emerged as a result of a putative recombination at the 5′ end of the S protein gene between CCoV-II and TGEV (Fig. 2). The CCoVIIa and IIb classifications are not officially accepted within CCoV taxonomy, but are widely cited in the literature [4].

Currently, CCoV-IIa exists in two biotypes that differ in pathogenicity and tissue tropism. The classical‖ CCoV-IIa is restricted to the small intestine, where it causes enteritis. In contrast, the emergent—pantropic CCoV-IIa biotype (prototypes CB/05 and 450/07)—can spread systemically, and has been detected by RT-PCR in various organs outside of the intestinal tract [11–15]. The genetic markers for pantropic CCoV-IIas are currently unknown.

The clinical signs associated with enteric CCoVs are not easily differentiated from those associated with other enteric pathogens. Consequently, CCoV diagnosis requires laboratory confirmation. PCR-based methods have been developed for detecting CCoV RNA in the feces of dogs and they are considered as the gold standard. A conventional RT-PCR test can detect alphacoronaviruses [16], and more specific PCR tests can be employed for further characterization into specific genotypes. It is particularly important since the two CCoV genotypes are commonly detected simultaneously in the same dog [2, 9, 17–21]. However, because of the highly variable nature of CCoV genomes, novel variants may be missed with this approach.

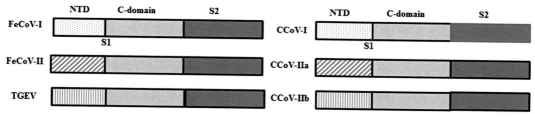

Fig. 2 Representation of the different domains present within the spike proteins of alpha-coronaviruses of cats (FCoV), dogs (CCoV), and pigs (TGEV). Adapted from Licitra et al. 2014. The different NTDs are filled to indicate homology and proposed recombination events across the species, with the remainder of S1 depicted in *light gray* and S2 in *dark gray*

2   Materials

2.1   Solutions

2.1.1   Tris-Ca²⁺ 0.01 M pH 7.2 Solution

For a 1000 mL solution, weight 1.21 g of Tris base ($C_4H_{11}NO_3$) (MW = 121.14) and dissolve in 800 mL deionized water using magnetic stirrer. Adjust pH to 7.2 with the appropriate volume of concentrated HCl. Add 0.02 g of $CaCl_2$ (MW = 110.98). Bring final volume to 1 L with deionized water. Autoclave and store at room temperature.

2.1.2   Tris-Borate-EDTA Buffer

1. Prepare a stock solution of EDTA 0.5 M pH 8.0:
   EDTA will not go completely into solution until the pH is adjusted to about 8.0. For a 500 mL stock solution of 0.5 M EDTA, weigh out 93.05 g ethylenediaminetetraacetic acid (EDTA) disodium salt (MW = 372.2). Dissolve in 400 mL deionized water and adjust the pH with NaOH. Top up the solution to a final volume of 500 mL. The solution is sterilized by autoclaving.

2. Prepare a stock solution of TBE 5×:
   Make a concentrated (5×) stock solution of TBE by weighing 54 g Tris base (MW = 121.14) and 27.5 g boric acid (FW = 1.83) and dissolving both in approximately 900 mL deionized water. Add 20 mL of 0.5 M EDTA (pH 8.0) and adjust the solution to a final volume of 1 L. This solution can be stored at room temperature but a precipitate will form in older solutions. Store the buffer in glass bottles and discard if a precipitate has formed.

3. Prepare a working solution of TBE
   For agarose gel electrophoresis, TBE can be used at a concentration of 0.5× (1:10 dilution of the concentrated stock). Dilute the stock solution by 10× in deionized water. Final solute concentrations are 45 mM Tris-borate and 1 mM EDTA. The buffer is now ready for use in running an agarose gel.

Table 1
Primers used for PCR amplification

Primer	Sequence (5′–3′)	Position	Amplicon size (bp)	CCoV type (gene)
CCV1 [16]	TCCAGATATGTAATGTTCGG	328–347[a]	410	I/II (M)
CCV2	TCTGTTGAGTAATCACCAGTC	717–737		
EL1F [17]	CAAGTTGACCGTCTTATTACTGGTAG	3538–3563[b]	346	I (S)
EL1R	TCATATACGTACCATTATAGCTGAAGA	3857–3883		
S5F [17]	TGCATTTGTGTCTCAGACTT	3486–3505[c]	694	IIa (S)
S6R	CCAAGGCCATTTTACATAAG	4160–4179		
CEPol-1 [19]	TCTACAATTATGGCTCTATCAC	20168–20190[d]	370	IIb (S)
TGSP-2	TAATCACCTAAMACCACATCTG	20516–20537		

[a]Primer position refers to the sequence of M gene of CCoV type IIa strain Insavc-1 (accession number D13096)
[b]Primer position refers to the sequence of S gene of CCoV type I strain Elmo/02 (accession number AY307020)
[c]Primer position refers to the sequence of S gene of CCoV type IIa strain Insavc-1 (accession number D13096).
[d]Primer position refers to the sequence of the complete genome of CCoV type IIb strain TGEV (accession number AJ271965-2)

2.1.3 *Ethidium Bromide*   Dissolve 0.2 g ethidium bromide to 20 mL water. Mix well and store in the dark (stock solution is 10 mg/mL concentration).

2.2 Oligonucleotides   The oligonucleotides for detection and characterization of CCoV strains are described in Table 1.

3 Methods

3.1 Collection of Fecal Samples

1. Fecal samples are collected from dogs using swabs.
2. The rectal swabs are placed in isothermal boxes using ice bags.
3. Transport the samples to the laboratory under refrigeration.
4. The feces should be kept at –20 °C until processed.

3.2 Preparation of 20 % Fecal Suspensions

1. In a centrifuge tube add 1–2 g of feces to prepare 20 % fecal suspension in Tris-Ca^{2+} (0.01 M, pH 7.2) buffer.
2. Mix by vortexing.
3. Centrifuge at $3000 \times g$ for 10 min.
4. Transfer the supernatant to another centrifuge tube.
5. Add 1/10 volume of chloroform.

6. Mix by vortexing.

7. Incubate at 4 °C for 10 min.

8. Centrifuge at $3000 \times g$ for 10 min.

9. Transfer the supernatant to 1.5 mL microcentrifuge tube.

10. Proceed to RNA extraction (*see* **Note 1**).

3.3 RNA Extraction (See Note 2)

1. Total RNA may be extracted from the supernatant fluid using a commercial RNA extraction kit following the manufacturer's instructions.

2. After RNA extraction it is recommended to proceed the cDNA synthesis in order to avoid RNA degradation.

3. For long-term storage of RNA store at −70 °C.

3.4 cDNA Synthesis

Reverse transcription (RT) may be carried out using random primers and reverse transcriptase enzyme according to the manufacturer's instructions (*see* **Note 3**).

3.5 PCR for CCoV Screening

To detect CCoV-I and CCoV-II, PCR may be performed with the CCV1-CCV2 primer pair which amplifies a 409 bp fragment of the gene encoding transmembrane protein M, as previously described [16]. The reagents for PCR reaction are described in Table 2.

1. Prepare the reaction mix as described in Table 2.

2. Distribute 40 µL of the reaction mix to each PCR tube.

3. Add 10 µL of cDNA to each tube for a final volume of 50 µL.

Table 2
Reagents used in PCR with primers CCV1/CCV2

Reagents	Volume (µL)
DNase/RNase-free dH_2O	27
10× PCR buffer	5
dXTP (dATP, dTTP, dCTP e dGTP) 2.5 mM	4
$MgCl_2$ 50 mM	1.5
CCV1 20 pmol	1
CCV2 20 pmol	1
Taq DNA polymerase(5 U/µL)	0.5
	40

4. PCR may be carried out in a DNA Thermal Cycler with the following reaction parameters: denaturation at 94 °C for 10 min followed by 35 cycles of (a) template denaturation at 94 °C for 1 min, (b) primer annealing at 55 °C for 1 min, and (c) extension at 72 °C 1 min, and complete the reaction with a single final extension step at 72 °C for 10 min.

5. Amplified products may be electrophoresed on 1.5 % (w/v) agarose gel in Tris-borate-EDTA (TBE) buffer at 80 V for about 90 min.

6. Visualize the DNA fragment by ethidium bromide staining under UV transillumination. A 100 bp DNA ladder can be used as size marker.

7. Samples that tested positive for CCoV may be subjected to direct sequencing.

8. The partial amplification of the gene M may be used to differentiate CCoV-I and CCoV-II strains based on the amino acid changes found in residues 127 (Ala → Ile/Ala → Val), 173 (Thr → Val), 193 (Met → Ile), 200 (Glu → Asp), and 201 (His → Asn) of the M protein [5, 21] (see **Note 4**).

9. To genotype/subtype CCoV strains or to diagnosis mixed CCoV infections it is necessary to amplify part of the S gene.

3.6 PCR for CCoV Genotyping/Subtyping

3.6.1 Differential Primers Directed to the Spike (S) Gene Should Be Used for CCoV Genotyping/ Subtyping as Follows

1. EL1F/EL1R (2611–2956): To amplify a 346 bp fragment corresponding to the S gene of the CCoV-I Elmo/02 strain (AY170345) [17].

2. S5F/S6R (3991–4684): To amplify a 694 bp product corresponding to the S gene of the CCoV-IIa Insavc strain (D13096) [17].

3. CEPol-1 and TGSp-2: To amplify a 370 bp product corresponding to nucleotides (nt) 20168–20537 of the TGEV Purdue genome (AJ271965.1) [19].

3.6.2 The Reagents for PCR Reaction Are Described in Table 3

1. Prepare the PCR mix as described in Table 3.

2. Distribute 20 μL of the reaction mix to each PCR tube.

3. Add 5 μL of cDNA to each tube for a final volume of 25 μL.

4. PCR may be carried out in a DNA Thermal Cycler with the reaction parameters provided in Table 4.

5. Amplified products may be electrophoresed on 1.5 % (w/v) agarose gel in TBE buffer at 80 V for about 90 min.

6. Visualize the DNA fragment by ethidium bromide staining under UV transillumination. A 100 bp DNA ladder can be used as size marker.

7. Samples that tested positive may be subjected to direct sequencing (see **Notes 5** and **6**).

Table 3
Reagents used in PCR to amplify the S gene

Reagents	Volume (µL)
DNase/RNase-free dH$_2$O	13.5
10× PCR buffer	2.5
dXTP (dATP, dTTP, dCTP e dGTP) 2.5 mM	2
MgCl$_2$ 50 mM	0.75
Forward Primer 20 pmol	0.5
Reverse Primer 20 pmol	0.5
Taq DNA polymerase (5 U/µL)	0.25
	20

Table 4
The reaction parameters for CCoV genotyping/subtyping

PCR conditions	Primer pair	
	EL1F/EL1R [17] S5F/S6R [17]	CEPol-1/TGSp-2 [19]
Denaturation at	94 °C for 10 min	95 °C for 5 min
	94 °C for 1 min	95 °C for 1 min
35 cycles	55 °C for 1 min	50 °C for 1 min
	72 °C 1 min	72 °C 1 min
Final extension at		72 °C for 10 min

3.7 Sequencing
(See Note 7)

1. The amplicons obtained after partial amplification of the M and S genes may be purified using commercial kits according to manufacturers' instructions.

2. After purification it is important to examine the DNA quality by using:

   (a) Agarose gel electrophoresis: purified DNA run as a single band.

   (b) Spectrophotometry : quantitate the amount of purified DNA by measuring the absorbance at 260 nm (the A260/A280 ratio should be 1.7–1.9).

3. The purified PCR products may be subjected to direct sequencing in both directions with the BigDye® Terminator v3.1 Cycle Sequencing Kit (Applied Biosystems™) according to standard protocols. Both strands of each amplicon should be sequenced at least twice.

3.8 Phylogenetic Analysis

1. For sequence comparisons the primer-binding sites should be excluded.

2. To perform the phylogenetic analysis, a database set containing sequences of CCoV-I, CCoV-IIa, and CCoV-IIb corresponding to the studied region should be retrieved from GenBank.

3. Nucleotide similarity with sequences deposited in the GenBank database may be assessed using the BLAST tool (http://blast.ncbi.nlm.nih.gov/Blast.cgi).

4. The sequences may be aligned with the BioEdit Sequence Alignment Editor v7.2.5(http://www.mbio.ncsu.edu/bioedit/bioedit.html).

5. The sequences should be subsequently analyzed using DAMBE software [22] to exclude identical sequences.

6. The Modeltest software 3.7 [23] may be used to test for a statistically justified model of DNA substitution that best fitted to the data set.

7. The evolutionary model should be selected and used for phylogenetic analysis.

8. Sequence analysis may be performed with the MEGA v.6.0 software [24].

9. For the construction of phylogenetic trees, deduced amino acid sequences should be used. Bootstrap analysis of 2000 replicates should be conducted to determine the significance of branching in the constructed tree.

4 Notes

1. If it is not possible to proceed RNA extraction keep the clarified suspension overnight at 4 °C. Long-term storage is not recommended.

2. Negative controls (fecal sample that tested positive for another enteric virus or fecal sample from normal dogs) and positive controls (CCoV-positive fecal sample or CCoV vaccine) should be included at every stage, from RNA extraction to PCR.

3. The advantages of using random hexamers instead of specific primers are as follows: It may give higher cDNA yield. The cDNA can be used in PCR assays specific for different viruses. It is a way of optimize the use of limited quantities of clinical sample.

4. This approach does not distinguish between single or multiple CCoVs in a dog or discriminate between IIa and IIb strains.

5. The conventional RT-PCR has high specificity and sensitivity and is a valuable diagnostic tool for the detection of CCoV in cases of single or multiple infections.

6. It is important to keep in mind the limitations of this methodology: It does not allow quantification of CCoV RNA in fecal samples which may be important in cases of multiple infections; another limitation is the inability to genotype divergent CCoVs that may not be amplified by the PCR primers.

7. Sequence analysis of the amplified fragment allows determining the types of CCoV circulating among dogs presenting mild or severe clinical signs of enteritis.

References

1. Adams MJ, Carstens EB (2012) Ratification vote on taxonomic proposals to the International Committee on Taxonomy of Viruses. Arch Virol 157:1411–1422

2. Pratelli A (2011) The evolutionary processes of canine coronavirus. Adv Virol 2011, 562831

3. Woo PC, Huang Y, Lau SK, Yuen KY (2010) Coronavirus genomics and bioinformatics analysis. Viruses 2:1804–1820

4. Licitra BN, Duhamel GE, Whittaker GR (2014) Canine enteric coronaviruses: emerging viral pathogens with distinct recombinant spike proteins. Viruses 6(8):3363–3376

5. Pratelli A, Martella V, Pistello M, Elia G, Decaro N, Buonavoglia D, Camero M, Tempesta M, Buonavoglia C (2003) Identification of coronaviruses in dogs that segregate separately from the canine coronavirus genotype. J Virol Methods 107:213–222

6. Pratelli A, Martella V, Elia G, Decaro N, Aliberti A, Buonavoglia D, Tempesta M, Buonavoglia C (2001) Variation of the sequence in the gene encoding for transmembrane protein M of canine coronavirus (CCV). Mol Cell Probes 15:229–233

7. Decaro N, Buonavoglia C (2008) An update on canine coronaviruses: viral evolution and pathobiology. Vet Microbiol 132:221–234

8. Pratelli A, Martella V, Decaro N, Tinelli A, Camero M, Cirone F, Elia G, Cavalli A, Corrente M, Greco G, Buonavoglia D, Gentile M, Tempesta M, Buonavoglia C (2003) Genetic diversity of a canine coronavirus detected in pups with diarrhoea in Italy. J Virol Methods 110:9–17

9. Decaro N, Mari V, Campolo M, Lorusso A, Camero M, Elia G, Martella V, Cordioli P, Enjuanes L, Buonavoglia C (2009) Recombinant canine coronaviruses related to transmissible gastroenteritis virus of swine are circulating in dogs. J Virol 83:1532–1537

10. Decaro N, Mari V EG et al (2010) Recombinant canine coronaviruses in dogs, Europe. Emerg Infect Dis 16(1):41–45

11. Decaro N, Martella V, Elia G, Addie DD, Camero M, Lucente MS, Martella V, Buonavoglia C (2007) Molecular characterization of the virulent canine coronavirus CB/05 strain. Virus Res 125(1):54–60

12. Decaro N, Mari V, Von Reitzenstein M, Lucente MS, Cirone F, Elia G, Martella V, King VL, Di Bello A, Varello K, Zhang S, Caramelli M, Buonavoglia C (2012) A pantropic canine coronavirus genetically related to the prototype isolate CB/05. Vet Microbiol 14:239–244

13. Ntafis V, Xylouri E, Mari V, Papanastassopoulou M, Papaioannou N, Thomas A, Buonavoglia C, Decaro N (2012) Molecular characterization of a canine coronavirus NA/09 strain detected in a dog's organs. Arch Virol 157:171–175

14. Zicola A, Jolly S, Mathijs E, Ziant D, Decaro N, Mari V, Thiry E (2012) Fatal outbreaks in dogs associated with pantropic canine coronavirus in France and Belgium. J Small Anim Pract 53:297–300

15. Pinto LD, Barros IN, Budaszewski RF, Weber MN, Mata H, Antunes JR, Boabaid FM, Wouters AT, Driemeier D, Brandão PE, Canal CW (2014) Characterization of pantropic canine coronavirus from Brazil. Vet J 202(3):659–662

16. Pratelli A, Tempesta M, Greco G, Martella V, Buonavoglia C (1999) Development of a nested PCR assay for the detection of canine coronavirus. J Virol Methods 80:11–15

17. Pratelli A, Decar N, Tinelli A, Martella V, Elia G, Tempesta M, Cirone F, Buonavoglia C (2004) Two genotypes of canine coronavirus simultaneously detected in fecal samples of dogs with diarrhea. J Clin Microbiol 42:1797–1799

18. Decaro N, Martella V, Ricci D, Elia G, Desario C, Campolo M, Cavaliere N, Di Trani L, Tempesta M, Buonavoglia C (2005) Genotype-specific fluorogenic RT-PCR assays for the detection and quantitation of canine coronavirus type I and type II RNA in faecal samples of dogs. J Virol Methods 130(1-2):72–78

19. Erles K, Brownlie J (2009) Sequence analysis of divergent canine coronavirus strains present in a UK dog population. Virus Res 141:21–25

20. Ntafis V, Mari V, Decaro N, Papanastassopoulou M, Pardali D, Rallis TS, Kanellos T, Buonavoglia C, Xylouri E (2013) Caninecoronavirus, Greece. Molecular analysis and genetic diversity characterization. Infect Genet Evol 16:129–136

21. Costa EM, Castro TX, Bottino FO, Cubel Garcia RCN (2014) Molecular characterization of canine coronavirus strains circulating in Brazil. Vet Microbiol 168:8–15

22. Xia X (2013) DAMBE5: a comprehensive software package for data analysis in molecular biology and evolution. Mol Biol Evol 30: 1720–1728

23. Posada D (2006) ModelTest Server: a web-based tool for the statistical selection of models of nucleotide substitution online. Nucleic Acids Res 34:W700–W703

24. Tamura K, Stecher G, Peterson D, Filipski A, Kumar S (2013) MEGA6: molecular evolutionary genetics analysis version 6.0. Mol Biol Evol 30:2725–2729

Part V

Next Generation Sequencing

Whole-Genome Sequencing of Porcine Epidemic Diarrhea Virus by Illumina MiSeq Platform

Leyi Wang, Tod Stuber, Patrick Camp, Suelee Robbe-Austerman, and Yan Zhang

Abstract

Porcine epidemic diarrhea virus (PEDV) belongs to the genus *Alphacoronavirus* of the family *Coronaviridae*. PEDV was identified as an emerging pathogen in US pig populations in 2013. Since then, this virus has been detected in at least 31 states in the USA and has caused significant economic loss to the swine industry. Active surveillance and characterization of PEDV are essential for monitoring the virus. Obtaining comprehensive information about the PEDV genome can improve our understanding of the evolution of PEDV viruses, and the emergence of new strains, and can enhance vaccine designs. In this chapter, both a targeted amplification method and a random-priming method are described to amplify the complete genome of PEDV for sequencing using the MiSeq platform. Overall, this protocol provides a useful two-pronged approach to complete whole-genome sequences of PEDV depending on the amount of virus in the clinical samples.

Key words Porcine epidemic diarrhea virus, Targeted amplification, SISPA, Whole-genome sequencing, MiSeq

1 Introduction

Complete genome sequencing and genetic analysis significantly improved our understanding of the evolution and relationship of porcine epidemic diarrhea virus (PEDV) strains worldwide. The first PEDV whole-genome sequence was completed for the prototype strain CV777 in 2001 [1]. Since then, several PEDV strains have been sequenced and now over 170 whole-genome sequences have been deposited in GenBank. Based on the phylogenetic analysis of the whole-genome sequence, PEDV has been classified into two Genogroups—1 and 2—which the variant and classical strains of US PEDV belong to, respectively [2].

Since the first 454 FLX pyrosequencing platform was introduced to the market in 2005, next-generation sequencing (NGS) has significantly advanced research in diverse fields. NGS has the

Leyi Wang (ed.), *Animal Coronaviruses*, Springer Protocols Handbooks, DOI 10.1007/978-1-4939-3414-0_18, © Springer Science+Business Media New York 2016

advantages of high-throughput and cost-effectiveness. Currently, there are several platforms available, including the Genome Analyser developed by Illumina/Solexa, and the Personal Genome Machine (PGM) by Ion Torrent. One of Illumina NGS platforms—MiSeq—is commonly used in diagnostic laboratories.

In general, sequencing viruses directly from fecal samples for PEDV are technically challenging without prior amplification with specific primers. In this chapter, we describe a useful two-pronged approach where the random-priming method can be used to sequence the complete PEDV genome from samples with Ct values of less than 15, whereas the targeted amplification method is recommended to be used to sequence clinical fecal samples with higher Ct values (low viral loads).

2   Materials

2.1   RNA Extraction from Feces or Intestinal Contents

1. MagMAX Pathogen RNA Kit (Life Technologies) for viral RNA extraction from fecal or intestinal contents (*see* **Note 1**).
2. HBSS (GIBCO).

2.2   Real-Time Reverse Transcriptase Polymerase Chain Reaction (RT-PCR) Reaction

1. One-Step RT-PCR kit (Qiagen).
2. Smart Cycler II (Cepheid, Sunnyvale CA).
3. 10 pmol Primers and probes [3] (*see* **Note 2**).

   Forward primer: 5′-CATGGGCTAGCTTTCAGGTC-3′.
   Reverse primer: 5′-CGGCCCATCACAGAAGTAGT-3′.
   Probe: 5′/56-FAM/CATTCTTGGTGGTCT   TTCAAT
   CCTGA/ZEN 3IABkFQ/3′.

2.3   Targeted Amplification One-Step RT-PCR

1. One-Step RT-PCR kit (Qiagen) (*see* **Note 3**).
2. Oligonucleotide primers dissolved in nuclease-free water to a stock concentration of 100 pmol/μl and a working concentration of 20 pmol/μl. The sequences for 19 pairs of primers are listed in Table 1.
3. Qiagen gel purification kit.
4. Qubit 2.0 Fluorometer (Life Technologies).

2.4   SISPA Method (Sequence-Independent, Single-Primer Amplification)

1. SuperScript III Reverse Transcriptase kit (Invitrogen).
2. RNase H treatment (NEB).
3. Klenow amplification (NEB).
4. Advantage 2 PCR kit (Clontech).
5. 10 mM dNTP mix (NEB).
6. RNase Inhibitor (Promega).

Table 1
Nineteen pairs of primers for whole-genome amplification of PEDV

Fragment no.	Sequence	Sense	Size
F1	ACTTAAAAAGATTTTCTATCTAC	Forward	1622
	CGTTAACGATACTAAGAGTGGC	Reverse	
F2	TGGTGACCTTGCAAGTGCAGC	Forward	1603
	ATTACCAACAGCCTTATTAAGC	Reverse	
F3	ACCATTGACCCAGTTTATAAGG	Forward	1587
	ACAAAGCACTTACAGTGGC	Reverse	
F4	TACACCTTTGATTAGTGTTGG	Forward	1614
	TTTGTAGCGTCTAACTCTAC	Reverse	
F5	GTACCAGGTGATCTCAATGTG	Forward	1615
	ACGTGGCAATGTCATGGACG	Reverse	
F6	ATGCTGCTGTTGCTGAGGCTC	Forward	1600
	TCAGTTGAGATAGAGTTGGC	Reverse	
F7	GTGACAAGTTCGTAGGCTC	Forward	1597
	TAAGTGACAGAACTCACAGG	Reverse	
F8	TGCACAAGGTCTTGTTAACATC	Forward	1601
	TCTGTGCACCATTAGGAGAATC	Reverse	
F9	ACCTGCGTGTAGTCAAGTGG	Forward	1599
	GTTACCAGTGGAACACCATC	Reverse	
F10	ACTGTGCCAACTTCAATACG	Forward	1611
	TCATCAACAAACACACCTGC	Reverse	
F11	TGCTCGCAGCATACTATGCAG	Forward	1588
	GTGGTGCAGGCAGCTGTTGAG	Reverse	
F12	TCTATGTGCACTAATTATGAC	Forward	1599
	TGATTGCACAATTCGGCCGC	Reverse	
F13	CCATACATGATTGCTTTGTC	Forward	1595
	ATCGTCAAGCAGGAGATCC	Reverse	
F14	TGTCTAGTAATGATAGCACG	Forward	1647
	TTATCCCATGTTATGCCGAC	Reverse	
F15	TAATGATGTTACAACAGGTCG	Forward	1554
	AAGCCATAGATAGTATACTTG	Reverse	
F16	TGAGTTGATTACTGGCACGCC	Forward	1598
	GTACTGTATGTAAAAACAGCAG	Reverse	

(continued)

Table 1
(continued)

Fragment no.	Sequence	Sense	Size
F17	ATCGCAATCTCAGCGTTATG	Forward	1596
	GTGTAAACTGCGCTATTACAC	Reverse	
F18	CTGCTTATTATAAGCATTAC	Forward	1603
	GCTTCTGCTGTTGCTTAAGC	Reverse	
F19	AGTCTCGTAACCAGTCCAAG	Forward	1065
	TTTTTTTTTTTTTGTGTATCCAT	Reverse	

7. Oligonucleotide primers [4] dissolved in nuclease-free water to a concentration of 50 μM, 1 μM, and 10 μM for P1, P2, and P3, respectively.

P1: GAC CAT CTA GCG ACC TCC ACN NNN NNN N.
P2: GAC CAT CTA GCG ACC TCC AC TTT TTTTTTT TTTTTTTT TT.
P3: GAC CAT CTA GCG ACC TCC AC.

8. QIAquick PCR Purification Kit (Qiagen).

2.5 Detection of PCR Products

1. Agarose.
2. Distilled water.
3. Ethidium bromide.
4. 1× TAE buffer: 40 mM Tris, 20 mM acetic acid, 1 mM EDTA.

2.6 Illumina Nextera DNA Library Preparation

1. Nextera XT Library Prep Kit 96 samples (Box 1 of 2) (Illumina).
2. Nextera XT Library Prep Kit 96 samples (Box 2 of 2) (Illumina).
3. Nextera XT Index Kit 96 indexes-192 samples.
4. Agencourt AMPure XP beads (Beckman Coulter).
5. 96-well PCR plate (Scientific Inc.).
6. 96 Deep Well Block (Invitrogen).
7. Microseal "B" adhesive seals (BioRad).
8. Magnetic plate stand-96 (Life, Technologies).
9. Ethanol, 200 proof (Sigma-Aldrich).

2.7 Next-Generation Sequencing

1. MiSeqv2 Reagent Kit 500 cycles PE-Box 1 of 2 (Illumina).
2. MiSeqv2 Reagent Kit Box 2 of 2 (Illumina).
3. MiSeq (Illumina).

2.8 Sequence Assembly and Analysis

1. Kraken.
2. Krona.
3. BWA—Burrows-Wheeler Alignment Tool.
4. SAMtools.
5. Picard.
6. BLAST.
7. BioPython.
8. GATK—Genome Analysis Toolkit.
9. R.
10. IGV.

3 Methods

3.1 Viral RNA Extraction

1. Fecal or intestinal contents were diluted in HBSS to a final concentration of 20 % and were homogenized by five stainless steel balls followed by a centrifuge step at 2000 RCF at 4 °C for 5 min.

2. The supernatant was used for RNA extraction by using the MagMAX Pathogen RNA/DNA Kit (Life Technologies) (*see* **Note 2**).

3.2 Real-Time RT-PCR Reaction

1. Real-time RT-PCR with a 25 μl reaction volume was completed using QIAGEN one-step RT-PCR kit: 5 μl 5× RT-PCR buffer, 0.5 μl forward primer (10 pmol), 0.5 μl reverse primer (10 pmol), 0.5 μl probe (10 pmol), 1 μl dNTP, 1 μl enzyme mix, 0.2 μl RNasin inhibitor (40 Unit/μl, Promega), and RNA temple: 2.5 μl.

2. The amplification conditions were 50 °C for 30 min; 95 °C for 15 min; and 45 cycles of 94 °C, 15 s, and 60 °C, 45 s.

3.3 One-Step RT-PCR Reaction

1. RT-PCR with a 25 μl reaction volume was completed using QIAGEN one-step RT-PCR kit: 5 μl 5× RT-PCR buffer, 0.8 μl forward primer (20 pmol), 0.8 μl reverse primer (20 pmol) (Table 1), 1 μl dNTP, 1 μl enzyme mix, 0.2 μl RNasin inhibitor (40 Unit/μl, Promega), and RNA temple: 2.5 μl.

2. The amplification conditions were 50 °C for 30 min; 95 °C for 15 min; and 45 cycles of 94 °C, 30 s, 54 °C, 30 s, and 72 °C, 1 min 30 s.

3. Analyze the PCR products on a 1 % agarose gel and migrate for 1 h at 90 V.

4. Excise the correct size bands and perform gel purification with a Qiagen gel purification kit (*see* **Note 4**).

5. Quantify the DNA generated by a fluorescence-based method (Qubit 2.0 Fluorometer) and final amount of DNA input as 1 μg (*see* **Note 5**).

3.4 SISPA Method (See Note 6)

3.4.1 First-Strand Synthesis

1. 1 μl of 50 μM random primer P1; 1 μl of 1 μM oligo dT primer P2; 1 μl 10 mM dNTP mix; 10 pg-5 μg of RNA template. Add water up to 13 μl total volume.

2. Incubate the reaction at 65 °C for 5 min and incubate on ice for at least 1 min.

3. Add 4 μl 5× first-strand buffer; 1 μl 0.1 M DTT; 1 μl RNase inhibitor; 1 μl of SuperScript III Reverse Transcriptase.

4. Incubate the reaction at 25 °C for 5 min, 50 °C for 30–60 min, and 70 °C for 15 min.

5. Add 1 μl RNase H (NEB) to the reaction.

6. Incubate at 37 °C for 20 min.

3.4.2 Klenow Amplification

1. Add 3 μl 10× Klenow reaction buffer; 1 μl of 25 μmol dNTP; and 1 μl of 1 μM random primer P1 to the reaction in Sect. 3.4.1.

2. Incubate at 95 °C for 2 min and cool to 4 °C.

3. Add 1 μl Klenow fragment (NEB).

4. Incubate at 37 °C for 60 min and 75 °C for 20 min.

3.4.3 PCR Amplification

1. 5 μl 10× Advantage 2 PCR buffer; 1 μl 50× dNTP mix; 2 μl 10 μM barcode primer P3; 1 μl 50× Advantage 2 Polymerase Mix; DNA template from Klenow amplification. Add water up to 50 μl total volume.

2. Incubate the reaction using the following PCR program: 1 cycle: 95 °C 5 min; 5 cycles: 95 °C 1 min; 59 °C 1 min; 68 °C 1 min 10 s; 33 cycles: 95 °C 20 s; 59 °C 20 s; 68 °C 1 min 30 s; 1 cycle: 68 °C 10 min.

3. Use 5 μl to analyze the PCR products on a 1 % agarose gel and migrate for 1 h at 90 V (*see* **Note 7**).

4. Use QIAquick PCR Purification Kit to purify the remaining 45 μl.

5. Quantify the DNA generated by a fluorescence-based method (Qubit 2.0 Fluorometer) and final amount of DNA input as 1 μg.

3.5 Library Preparation Using Nextera XT Kit

1. Perform the library preparation based on the Illumina company manual, which includes tagmentation of genomic DNA, PCR amplification, PCR cleanup, library normalization, and final library pooling for MiSeq sequencing.

3.6 Sequence Assembly and Analysis

1. Kraken is used to initially identify raw reads and provide a graphical representation of the reads using Krona. A custom Kraken database is used. It was built using the standard database containing all Ref Seq bacteria and virus genomes along with all complete swine enteric coronavirus disease (SECD) genomes available at NCBI and a pig genome.

2. Raw reads are run through an in-house custom shell script. In brief, 18 complete genomes from NCBI representing the 4 SECD virus species (TGEV, PRCV, PEDV, and PDCoV) are used as references to align raw reads. A function is looped 3×. This function aligns and removes duplicates, creates a VCF, updates reference with VCF information, and performs a BLAST search against the nt database using the updated reference. Eighteen complete genomes are used to start the initial loop. From this first loop the top hit returned is used as the reference for the next loop. A total of three loops are performed to find the best reference.

3. After the best reference has been found, alignment metrics including read counts, mean depth of coverage, and percent of genome with coverage are collected.

4. Reports summarizing the alignment metrics (Fig. 1) along with Kraken identification interactive Krona HTML file, a FASTA of assembled genome, and depth of coverage profile graph (Fig. 2) are e-mailed to concerned individuals.

5. The assembled FASTA file can be visually verified in IGV using the BAM and VCF output from the script. If necessary the FASTA can be corrected in program of choice.

6. Script details are provided on GitHub (https://github.com/USDA-VS/public/blob/master/secd/idvirus.sh).

```
Sample: OH851-RP-Virus
Reference_Set: SECD
R1 file size: 451M, read count: 914188
R2 file size: 451M, read count: 914188
223,955 virus reads --> 24.4977% of total reads

Alignment stats (reference guided):
reference used                              read count  percent cov  ave depth
Porcine_epidemic_diarrhea_virus-KJ399978      346,926      98.36%      2,764X
Porcine_Resp_Corona_Virus-DQ811787             68,978      50.83%        713X
---------------------------------------------------
*** NT Database ***
query ID                                    qlength  slength  % id   mis  evalue  bscore  Description
Porcine_epidemic_diarrhea_virus-KJ399978     28025    28029   99.98   1    0.0     51729  Porcine epidemic diarrhea virus strain OH851, complete genome KJ399978.1
Porcine_Resp_Corona_Virus-DQ811787           26617    27550   93.00 1654    0.0     38778  PRCV ISU-1, complete genome DQ811787.1
```

Fig. 1 Report summary for sample OH851-RP-Virus. The reference set used to initiate the shell script was SECD (swine enteric coronavirus diseases). File size and read counts for each fastq file are shown. Provided by Kraken, 223,955 virus reads were identified. "Reference used" is the closest finding in the NCBI nt database. The read count shows the number of raw reads shown to match the reference. "Percent cov" shows the percent of reference having coverage. A coverage of 98.36 % for PEDV indicates a true find relative to the sporadic <51 % coverage seen from PRCV, although in this case, the presence of PRCV cannot be ruled out. There were no reads matching TGEV and PDCoV, which were not shown. Because of the high percent of genome coverage, the completed reference-guided assembly for PEDV was BLAST against the nt database to provide mismatches, *e*-value, and bit score against the most closely related publicly available genome

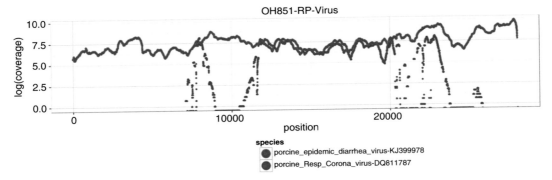

Fig. 2 The depth of coverage profiles for sample OH851-RP-Virus. The *x*-axis is the genome position. The *y*-axis is the log depth of coverage. Reads matching any of the four SECD target viral species are shown

4   Notes

1. The MagMAX Pathogen RNA/DNA Kit was used for the extraction of nucleic acid for pathogen detection—including the detection of TGEV, PEDV, and PDCoV—from pig feces or intestinal contents.

2. The real-time RT-PCR assay was developed by our laboratory and the primers and probes target the M gene of the virus.

3. In our laboratory, the QIAGEN one-step RT-PCR kit has been used to amplify RT-PCR products between 100 bp and 1.8 kb in length.

4. Alternatively, 5 µl out of 25 µl could be loaded on the gel to confirm that each target band is amplified and then the remaining 20 µl can be purified by QIAquick PCR Purification Kit.

5. A smaller amount of input DNA than the required 1 µg for targeted amplification method could be used to avoid overwhelming sequence reads.

6. The SISPA method is recommended when the Ct value of real-time RT-PCR is below 15.

7. When 5 µl was applied to the gel, a smear bank can be observed.

References

1. Kocherhans R, Bridgen A, Ackermann M, Tobler K (2001) Completion of the porcine epidemic diarrhoea coronavirus (PEDV) genome sequence. Virus Genes 23:137–144

2. Wang L, Byrum B, Zhang Y (2014) New variant of porcine epidemic diarrhea virus, United States, 2014. Emerg Infect Dis 20:917–919

3. Wang L, Zhang Y, Byrum B (2014) Development and evaluation of a duplex real-time RT-PCR for detection and differentiation of virulent and variant strains of porcine epidemic diarrhea viruses from the United States. J Virol Methods 207:154–157

4. Victoria JG, Kapoor A, Dupuis K, Schnurr DP, Delwart EL (2008) Rapid identification of known and new RNA viruses from animal tissues. PLoS Pathog 4:e1000163

Chapter 19

Next-Generation Sequencing for Porcine Coronaviruses

Douglas Marthaler, Ann Bohac, Aaron Becker, and Nichole Peterson

Abstract

The outbreak of porcine epidemic diarrhea virus and the discovery of porcine deltacoronavirus in the USA have led to multiple questions about the evolution of coronaviruses in swine. Coronaviruses are enveloped virus, containing a positive-sense single-stranded RNA genome (26–30 kb) that can cause respiratory or enteric illness in swine. With current technologies, the complete viral genomes can be determined to understand viral diversity and evolution. In this chapter, we describe a method to deep genome sequence porcine coronavirus on the Illumina MiSeq, avoiding the number of contaminating reads associated with the host and other microorganisms.

Key words Porcine coronaviruses, Next-generation sequencing, Whole-genome sequencing, Porcine epidemic diarrhea virus, Porcine deltacoronavirus

1 Introduction

Coronaviruses (CoVs) have negatively impacted the health of pigs for multiple decades [1]. Currently, five swine CoVs have been identified: transmissible gastroenteritis virus (TGEV), porcine respiratory coronavirus (PRCV), porcine epidemic diarrhea virus (PEDV), hemagglutinating encephalomyelitis virus (HEV), and porcine deltacoronavirus (PDCoV) [2, 3]. Multiple studies have described methods to detect CoVs by PCR methods [4–7]. In addition, multiple manuscripts have described Sanger sequencing methodologies to investigate the genetic diversity and evolution of individual or partial CoV genes [7–9]. However, investigating partial genome of these CoVs underestimates the evolutionary history of these viruses [10].

In the pursuit to investigate recombinant regions within the CoV genome and to further enhance our understanding of CoV evolution, CoV genome sequencing has become very valuable. In addition, next-generation sequencing (NGS) technology has facilitated the use of complete genomic sequencing with extreme high coverage and reduced the cost compared to Sanger sequencing.

Leyi Wang (ed.), *Animal Coronaviruses*, Springer Protocols Handbooks,
DOI 10.1007/978-1-4939-3414-0_19, © Springer Science+Business Media New York 2016

Many laboratories have purchased desktop NGS sequencers to expand their sequencing capabilities, due to the relatively low cost associated with the equipment. However, achieving viral genomes directly from samples can be difficult since the total RNA, including mRNA from host cells and bacteria, is also sequenced [11–13]. Nevertheless, NGS technology is a very powerful tool in generating CoV genomes, which could lead to a better understanding of CoV evolution.

2 Materials

2.1 Sample Handling and RNA Extraction

1. Phosphate-buffered solution (PBS).
2. Stomacher® 400 Circulator (Laboratory Supply Network, USA).
3. 1 mL Syringe without needle.
4. 0.22 μm Syringe filters.
5. Turbo DNA (Thermo Fisher Scientific, USA).
6. RNase ONE™ Ribonuclease (Promega, USA).
7. MagMAX™-96 Viral RNA Isolation Kit (Thermo Fisher Scientific, USA). Store the buffers at room temperature, the RNA-binding beads at 4 °C, and carrier RNA and binding enhancer at –20 °C.

2.2 Evaluation and Assessment of RNA Mass Using Ribogreen and Agilent Bioanalyzer

1. Quant-iT™ RiboGreen® RNA Assay Kit (Life Technologies, USA).
2. FLx800 Fluorescence Reader or similar UV-V reader (Bio-Tek, USA).
3. λ RNA Standard (Life Technologies, USA).
4. Black 96-well plate (Thermo Fisher Scientific, USA).
5. Agilent RNA 6000 Nano kit (Agilent, USA).
6. Molecular-grade water (Sigma-Aldrich, USA).

2.3 Illumina TruSeq RNA Library Creation and Validation

1. TruSeq RNA Sample Preparation Kit, Box A (Illumina, USA).
2. TruSeq RNA Sample Preparation Kit, Box B (Illumina, USA).
3. TruSeq RNA Sample Preparation Kit, PCR Prep Box (Illumina, USA).
4. SuperScript II (Life Technologies, USA).
5. AmPure XP beads (Beckman Coulter, USA).
6. Ethanol, 200 proof (Sigma-Aldrich, USA).
7. Microseal "B" adhesive seals (BioRad, USA).
8. RNase/DNase-free strip tubes and caps.
9. Thermal Scientific PCR plates (Life Technologies, USA).

10. BioRad PCR plates (BioRad, USA).

11. Magnetic plate or stand (Life Technologies, USA).

12. Qiagen EB Buffer (Qiagen, USA).

2.4 Sequencing on the Illumina Miseq

1. MiSeq Reagent Kit v2 (Illumina, USA).

2. PhiX Control (Illumina, USA).

3. 2 nM Normalized libraries.

4. Stock 1.0 N NaOH (Illumina, USA).

5. Tris-Cl, 10 mM, pH 8.5 (Qiagen, USA).

2.5 Sequence Assembly

1. Trimmomatic.

2. DNASTAR software package.

3 Methods

3.1 Sample Handling and RNA Extraction

1. Fecal swabs: Place the swab into a tube containing 2 mL of PBS. Vortex the sample in the solution for 30 s. Centrifuge the sample for 20 min at $3000 \times g$. Transfer the supernatant to a new tube, and store the sample at -80 °C.

2. Feces: Weigh 1 g of feces and place the feces into a tube containing 3 mL of PBS. Vortex the sample in the solution for 30 s. Centrifuge the sample for 20 min at $3000 \times g$. Transfer the supernatant to a new tube, and store the sample at -80 °C.

3. Tissues: Weigh 1 g of the tissue and place the gram in 3 mL of PBS. Homogenize the tissue for 1 min. Transfer the supernatant to a new tube, and centrifuge the sample for 20 min at $3000 \times g$. Transfer the supernatant to a new tube, and store the sample at -80 °C.

4. Using a syringe, aspirate the supernatant from each sample and pass the sample through a 0.22 μm filter into a new tube (*see* **Note 1**).

5. After the samples have been filtered, in a separate tube add:

   (a) 20 μL of 10× Turbo DNase Buffer.

   (b) 12 μL of Turbo DNase.

   (c) 2 μL of RNase ONE Ribonuclease.

   (d) 200 μL of filtered sample.

6. Mix the sample and reagents gently with the pipette or lightly vortex mixture.

7. Incubate the samples for 37 °C for 90 min, and immediately proceed to the extraction to inactivate the DNase and RNase.

8. Extract the RNA from the treated samples using the MagMAX™-96 Viral RNA Isolation Kit. Store the extracted RNA (40 μL) at -80 °C.

3.2 Evaluation and Assessment of RNA Mass Using Ribogreen and Agilent Bioanalyzer

1. Quantify the RNA using the Quant-iT™ RiboGreen® RNA Assay Kit, according to the manufacturer's instructions (*see* **Note 2**).

2. Once the concentration of RNA has been determined, assess the RNA integrity using the Agilent Bioanalyzer, according to the manufacturer's instructions (*see* **Note 3**).

3.3 Illumina TruSeq RNA Library Creation and Validation

1. Follow the manufacturer's protocol for TruSeq RNA Library Preparation Kit v2 as recommended, with the following modification (*see* **Note 4**).

2. Normalize Ribogreen quantitated RNA samples to 20 ng/μL with water, for an input mass of 100 ng per reaction. If starting RNA of 20 ng/μL is unavailable, use a maximum of 5 μL purified sample to start the elute, prime, and fragment steps.

3. Shorten RNA fragmentation time to 2 min to keep the fragments as long as possible to take advantage of the sequencing length obtained using MiSeq 2×250 bp run.

4. Validate the library yield using a fluorometric assay, either PicoGreen or Qubit, according to the manufacturer's instructions (*see* **Note 5**).

5. Normalize libraries to 10 nM using Qiagen EB buffer or standard Tris buffer. If final undiluted library concentrations are below 10 nM, normalize to 2 nM.

3.4 Sequencing on the Illumina MiSeq

1. Combine equal volumes of 10 or 2 nM normalized libraries depending on the type of MiSeq run required for sample number.

2. Denature and dilute libraries to 8 pM for sequencing with 1 % PhiX spike.

3. Sequence pooled libraries using a MiSeq Nano 250 bp PE (MiSeq 500 cycle v2 Nano) run if sequencing less than two libraries (*see* **Note 6**).

4. Load instrument according to the manufacturer's specifications.

3.5 Sequence Assembly (See Note 7)

1. Transfer the fastq from the MiSeq machine. The fastq files will need to undergo a quality assurance to remove adapter sequences and low-quality read, which can be done with Trimmomatic, an open-source software[14] (*see* **Note 8**).

2. Reference-based assembly for coronavirus genomes.

   (a) Open the SeqManNGen program, select reference-based assembly, and load the reference CoV genome and the correlating paired fastq files to the sample and run the assembly.

   (b) Evaluate assembly of reads (*see* **Note 9**). If there are regions with minimal coverage, this indicates that the reads do not match the reference sequence. Remove the reference strain and split the contig at the low-coverage regions. Trim the 5′ and 3′ regions of the new contigs at the split region.

(c) Preform reference-based assembly with the newly generated contigs. The contig ends will extend with the viral reads.

(d) Merge the contigs together to generate a single contig.

(e) Remap the reads to the contig to verify accurate generation of the viral genome and sufficient coverage. The contig can be saved as a fasta file for future phylogenetic analysis.

3. De novo assembly for viral genomes.

(a) Open the SeqManNGen program, select reference-based assembly, and load the Susscrofa genome and the correlating paired fastq files to the sample. In the advance options, select saved unmapped reads, which will save the reads that did not map to Sus scrofa genome once the assembly has finished. Run the assembly.

(b) After the program finished running, open SeqManNGen program again, select de novo assembly, and load the unassembled fastq file from the previous reference-based assembly.

(c) Once the de novo assembly has finished, BLAST the contigs to locate the designated coronavirus contigs.

(d) Remap the reads to the coronavirus sequence and verify accurate and sufficient coverage. The contig can be saved as a fasta file for future phylogenetic analysis.

4 Notes

1. Some samples may contain excess organic material and clog the filter. If this occurs, centrifuge the sample for another 20 min at $3000 \times g$.

2. Quantification needs to occur with a fluorometry system that measures only single-stranded nucleic acids and is insensitive to organic contaminants commonly used in extraction kits, which allows for more accurate quantification of input mass and higher probability of successful library preparation.

3. The RNA sample needs to be assessed for the concentration of host ribosomal RNA (rRNA). This assessment does not remove host rRNA, but ensures that the RNA is free of rRNA, which severely dilutes the number of viral reads (Fig. 1).

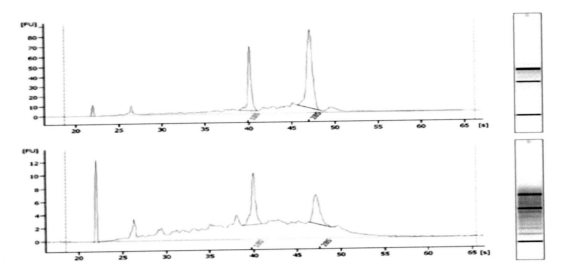

Fig. 1 Example of rRNA contamination. The Agilent traces are indicative of incomplete viral RNA purification with 18S and 28S host rRNA peaks

4. The mRNA purification strategy should be skipped since the oligo-dT-coated magnetic beads were used to specifically bind poly-A-tailed mRNA. The viral RNA will not be poly-A tailed. Start the library preparation at step "Incubate RFP," which is the start of random primed cDNA synthesis.

5. Typical concentrations of viral RNA libraries for the TruSeq RNA library preparation kit are 1–15 ng/μL.

6. The concentration of coronavirus must be estimated by RT-PCR. However, the concentration by RT-PCR may not indicate successful generation of the complete viral genome since total RNA was used in the library preparation. Generally, lower concentration of viral particles by RT-PCR indicates that more reads are needed to generate a complete genome. If libraries have limited host contamination and have an acceptable concentration of viral RNA (Ct value <25), a 1 million read output per sample should be sufficient for assembly. If more reads are needed per sample, the MiSeq v2 250 PE kit can be used.

7. Two major assembly methodologies are available, reference based and de novo assembly. However, due to the genetic diversity of viruses, gaps in coverage can occur during reference-based assembly. We will briefly discuss both options in this chapter. Reference-based assembly maps the MiSeq reads to a known sequence (template) to build a contig while de novo assembly does not use a sequence to build a contig, which take longer to run. Since the MiSeq generates reads from total RNA, host reads need to be removed to facilitate de novo assembly, which can be done by first mapping the reads to the swine genome and saving the unmapped reads. Hence, the de

novo assembly process described here first utilizes a reference-based assembly (to remove host reads) and then a de novo assembly to construct contigs.

8. Many different programs are available to remove adapter sequences and low-quality read and assembly genomes, and each program uses slightly different algorithms and operations to accomplish this task. Removing low-quality reads is necessary before attempting viral assembly.

9. Coverage across the genome will vary and is expected. The valleys, which indicate less coverage, should have approximately the same amount of coverage (Fig. 2a). If valleys with less coverage are comparable to the other valleys with high coverage, the reads did not match to the reference due to genetic diversity of the CoV strain (Fig. 2b).

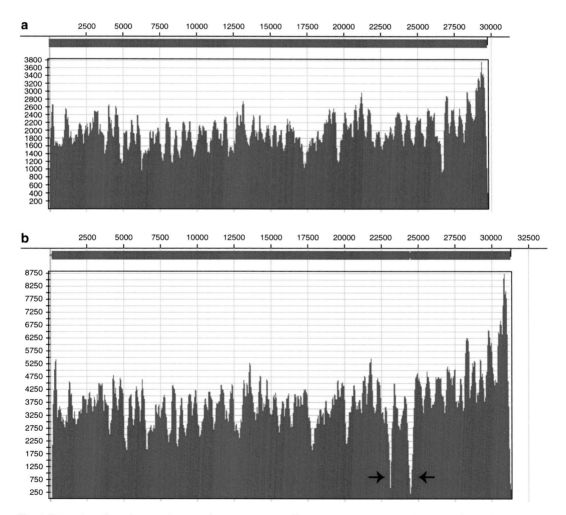

Fig. 2 Examples of reads mapping to reference genome. The *x*-axis represents the length of the genome while the *y*-axis represents depth of coverage. (**a**) Unequal coverage across the genome. (**b**) Gaps in coverage due to genetic differences between the reference genome and sequenced sample, indicated by the *black arrows*

References

1. Saif L, Pensaert MB, Sestak K, Yeo S, Jung K (2012) Diseases of swine. In: Zimmerman JJ, Ebrary I (eds) Coronaviruses, 10th edn. Wiley-Blackwell, Chichester, West Sussex, pp 501–524

2. Masters P, Perlman S (2013) Fields virology. In: Fields BN, Knipe DM, Howley PM, Ebrary I (eds) Coronaviridae, 6th edn. Wolters Kluwer Health/Lippincott Williams & Wilkins, Philadelphia, pp 825–858

3. Woo PC, Lau SK, Lam CS, Lau CC, Tsang AK, Lau JH, Bai R, Teng JL, Tsang CC, Wang M, Zheng BJ, Chan KH, Yuen KY (2012) Discovery of seven novel Mammalian and avian coronaviruses in the genus deltacoronavirus supports bat coronaviruses as the gene source of alphacoronavirus and betacoronavirus and avian coronaviruses as the gene source of gammacoronavirus and deltacoronavirus. J Virol 86:3995–4008. doi:10.1128/JVI.06540-11

4. Marthaler D, Raymond L, Jiang Y, Collins J, Rossow K, Rovira A (2014) Rapid detection, complete genome sequencing, and phylogenetic analysis of porcine deltacoronavirus. Emerg Infect Dis 20:1347–1350. doi:10.3201/eid2008.140526

5. Zhao J, Shi BJ, Huang XG, Peng MY, Zhang XM, He DN, Pang R, Zhou B, Chen PY (2013) A multiplex RT-PCR assay for rapid and differential diagnosis of four porcine diarrhea associated viruses in field samples from pig farms in East China from 2010 to 2012. J Virol Methods 194:107–112. doi:10.1016/j.jviromet.2013.08.008

6. Rodriguez E, Betancourt A, Relova D, Lee C, Yoo D, Barrera M (2012) Development of a nested polymerase chain reaction test for the diagnosis of transmissible gastroenteritis of pigs. Rev Sci Tech 31:1033–1044

7. Costantini V, Lewis P, Alsop J, Templeton C, Saif LJ (2004) Respiratory and fecal shedding of porcine respiratory coronavirus (PRCV) in sentinel weaned pigs and sequence of the partial S-gene of the PRCV isolates. Arch Virol 149:957–974. doi:10.1007/s00705-003-0245-z

8. Li R, Qiao S, Yang Y, Su Y, Zhao P, Zhou E, Zhang G (2014) Phylogenetic analysis of porcine epidemic diarrhea virus (PEDV) field strains in central China based on the ORF3 gene and the main neutralization epitopes. Arch Virol 159:1057–1065. doi:10.1007/s00705-013-1929-7

9. Sun R, Leng Z, Zhai SL, Chen D, Song C (2014) Genetic variability and phylogeny of current Chinese porcine epidemic diarrhea virus strains based on spike, ORF3, and membrane genes. Sci World J 2014:208439. doi:10.1155/2014/208439

10. Vlasova AN, Marthaler D, Wang Q, Culhane MR, Rossow KD, Rovira A, Collins J, Saif LJ (2014) Distinct characteristics and complex evolution of PEDV strains, North America, May 2013-February 2014. Emerg Infect Dis 20:1620–1628. doi:10.3201/eid2010.140491

11. Belak S, Karlsson OE, Blomstrom AL, Berg M, Granberg F (2013) New viruses in veterinary medicine, detected by metagenomic approaches. Vet Microbiol 165:95–101. doi:10.1016/j.vetmic.2013.01.022

12. Hall RJ, Wang J, Todd AK, Bissielo AB, Yen S, Strydom H, Moore NE, Ren X, Huang QS, Carter PE, Peacey M (2014) Evaluation of rapid and simple techniques for the enrichment of viruses prior to metagenomic virus discovery. J Virol Methods 195:194–204. doi:10.1016/j.jviromet.2013.08.035

13. Shah JD, Baller J, Zhang Y, Silverstein K, Xing Z, Cardona CJ (2014) Comparison of tissue sample processing methods for harvesting the viral metagenome and a snapshot of the RNA viral community in a turkey gut. J Virol Methods 209:15–24. doi:10.1016/j.jviromet.2014.08.011

14. Bolger AM, Lohse M, Usadel B (2014) Trimmomatic: a flexible trimmer for Illumina sequence data. Bioinformatics 30:2114–2120. doi:10.1093/bioinformatics/btu170

INDEX

Leyi Wang (ed.), *Animal Coronaviruses*, Springer Protocols Handbooks,
DOI 10.1007/978-1-4939-3414-0, © Springer Science+Business Media New York 2016

Printed in the United States
By Bookmasters